DEC 0 2 2015
W9-CEK-458
John C. Fremont Branch Library
6121 Melrose Avenue
Los Angeles, CA 90038

yoga therapy *for* stress & anxiety

DEC 1 0 2015

Robert Butera, PhD ❀ *Erin Byron, MA* ❀ *Staffan Elgelid, PhD, PT*

yoga therapy *for* stress & anxiety

Create a Personalized Holistic Plan to Balance Your Life

Llewellyn Publications
Woodbury, Minnesota

613.71
B983-1

22222 7820

Yoga Therapy for Stress and Anxiety: Create a Personalized Holistic Plan to Balance Your Life © 2015 by Robert Butera, PhD, Erin Byron, MA, and Staffan Elgelid, PhD, PT. All rights reserved. No part of this book may be used or reproduced in any manner whatsoever, including Internet usage, without written permission from Llewellyn Publications, except in the case of brief quotations embodied in critical articles and reviews.

First Edition
First Printing, 2015

Cover art: iStockphoto.com / 12506613 / GlobalStock
Cover design: Teresa Pojar
Interior illustrations: Mary Ann Zapalac

Llewellyn is a registered trademark of Llewellyn Worldwide Ltd.

Library of Congress Cataloging-in-Publication Data
Butera, Robert, 1964–
Yoga therapy for stress and anxiety : create a personalized holistic plan to balance your life / Robert Butera, Erin Byron, and Staffan Elgelid.
pages cm
ISBN 978-0-7387-4575-6
1. Hatha yoga—Therapeutic use. 2. Stress management. 3. Anxiety—Treatment. I. Byron, Erin, 1973– II. Elgelid, Staffan. III. Title.
RM727.Y64B89 2015
613.7'046—dc23
2015020532

Llewellyn Worldwide Ltd. does not participate in, endorse, or have any authority or responsibility concerning private business transactions between our authors and the public.

All mail addressed to the author is forwarded but the publisher cannot, unless specifically instructed by the author, give out an address or phone number.

Any Internet references contained in this work are current at publication time, but the publisher cannot guarantee that a specific location will continue to be maintained. Please refer to the publisher's website for links to authors' websites and other sources.

Llewellyn Publications
A Division of Llewellyn Worldwide Ltd.
2143 Wooddale Drive
Woodbury, MN 55125-2989
www.llewellyn.com

Printed in the United States of America

Other Books by Robert Butera, PhD

The Pure Heart of Yoga:
Ten Essential Steps for Personal Transformation (2009)

Meditation for Your Life: Creating a Plan that Suits Your Style (2012)

Forthcoming Books by Robert Butera, PhD, and Erin Byron, MA

Llewellyn's Complete Book of Mindful Living:
Awareness & Meditation Practices for Living in the Present Moment (2016)

Contents

Exercise List

Part I

Chapter 1

Chapter 2

Chapter 3

Chapter 4

Part II

Chapter 5

Chapter 6

Chapter 7

Chapter 8

Chapter 9

Part III

Chapter 10

List of Yoga Postures

Part I

Chapter 1

Chapter 3

Part II

Chapter 5

The practices, movements, and methods described in this book should not be used as an alternative to professional diagnosis or treatment. The authors and publisher of this book are not responsible in any manner whatsoever for any injury or negative effects which might occur through following the instructions and advice contained in this book. It is recommended that before beginning any treatment or exercise program, you should consult medical professionals to determine whether you should undertake this course of practice.

Foreword

Authors' Stories

Bob Butera, PhD, is influenced by his grandparents' strong faith and community service and his parents' willingness to permit him to study yoga as his academic concentration at the university level when there was no apparent career potential. The discipline required to participate in a variety of competitive athletics ultimately helped Bob have a love and understanding of how the body and mind work together. Bob was introduced to meditation via martial arts in the United States, Japan, and Taiwan as a college student. Yoga study began during college in the 1980s. Bob experienced one-on-one intensive yoga training at the Yoga Institute, where he lived for six months in 1989. This led to a religious awakening and he achieved a Master of Divinity degree at the Earlham School of Religion before completing his PhD in yoga therapy at the California Institute of Integral Studies. For the past twenty-five years he has served as a Comprehensive Yoga Therapist and trainer of yoga therapists, yoga teachers, and meditation instructors. He is author of *The Pure Heart of Yoga* (2009) and *Meditation for Your Life* (2012).

Erin Byron, MA, is a psychotherapist whose Master of Arts dissertation was "Yoga for Post-Traumatic Stress Disorder." It was during this study that Erin met Bob and has since enjoyed a long mentoring and working relationship with him. Erin and Bob, along with Kristen

Butera, Staffan Elgelid, and other senior yoga professionals created Comprehensive Yoga Therapist Training. Erin is the director of Welkin YogaLife Institute in Brantford, Ontario, Canada, where she trains yoga and meditation teachers and Comprehensive Yoga Therapists. Erin enjoys traveling to teach these subjects as well as leading diverse groups such as university students, business professionals, and mental health practitioners on topics such as body psychology, transforming feelings, yoga therapy, and yoga for mental health issues such as depression, anxiety, and post-traumatic stress.

Staffan Elgelid, PhD, PT, GCFP, is associate professor of physical therapy and the co-chair of the Health and Wellness Initiative at Nazareth College in Rochester, New York. He also maintains a practice of Feldenkrais and yoga therapy clients. Staffan came to the United States from Sweden in 1980 and earned his Bachelor of Science in physical therapy, allowing him to open a private practice that focused on PT for athletes. He worked with athletes and teams at events such as the World Championship in Track and Field, the Boston Marathon, the Berlin Marathon, and the New York Marathon. Staffan lectures at conferences on a wide variety of topics, including integrative medicine, mentoring, visualization, strength training, health and wellness, evidenced-based medicine, as well as SmartCore training, which he produced a video about. In addition to his PT degree Staffan is a certified Feldenkrais teacher. He has been on the board of the North American Feldenkrais Guild, served as the North American representative for the International Feldenkrais Federation, and is on the advisory board of the International Association of Yoga Therapists (IAYT) as well as a peer reviewer for the IAYT journal and several other peer-reviewed academic publications.

Please see our acknowledgements at the back of the book to learn more about those who have supported us on this journey.

Introduction

It seems like everyone these days is coping with a great deal of stress. Some people would say they have had anxiety arise briefly and others have lived with it daily for a long time. Whether you suffer from the occasional stress or have been dealing with profound anxiety, this book offers you a personalized approach to recovering from anxiety and transforming stress into ease. You don't even have to be experienced in yoga—this book is written with the average reader in mind! This book is for all of you, no matter your age, beliefs, or physical fitness. Through effective yoga philosophy and practices, practical exercises, and clear reflection questions, we guide you through the process of self-understanding to remove stress and anxiety from your emotions, mind, and life.

Imagine that you, and each human being, are like an ecosystem—a self-contained environmental system such as a pond. An ecosystem has many intricate parts. Even something as small as a pond relies on a water source such as rain, runoff, or an underground spring. In this pond are all types of grasses, moss, algae, and a variety of microorganisms that exist in perfect balance because of the bugs who consume some of grasses. To keep perfect harmony the bugs attract fish, bats, and birds. Turtles, frogs, and occasionally larger birds of prey like herons and eagles are also integral parts of this ecosystem. The sun heats the water, the winter freezes it. Over the years the mud collects silt from the rains. The cycle continues as decaying plant material regenerates life.

Imagine taking away any one of these elements. Take away the grass and the mud will overflow the banks, the shore will erode, the baby fish will have nowhere to hide, and soon the ecosystem will be shot. Remove the insects and the fish, bats, birds, frogs, and turtles will disappear. Take away the wind or underground stream and the pond becomes a dry creek.

We human beings are complex ecosystems. Throw any part of ourselves out of balance and you will end up with a stressed person, just like an ecosystem can be stressed from factors such as climate change, invasive plants, or other calamity. You exist via the air you breathe, the food you eat, the people you know, the work you do, the thoughts you think, the dreams you have, your hobbies, your education, and so on; you are a magnificent coalescence of all the things that make up life. Throw off one part of your life and just like the pond, you will feel off-kilter.

The beauty of all this is that an ecosystem is constantly recovering balance. Some years there are more bugs, or grasses, or fish, but the endeavor toward balance is always there. If your stress or anxiety seems overwhelming right now, the good news is that if you are reading this book you are alive and your ecosystem is functioning! Principles and practices of Comprehensive Yoga Therapy will help it be as optimal as possible. This book is designed to give you tools to maintain balance.

What Is Comprehensive Yoga Therapy?

Comprehensive Yoga Therapy is a specific kind of yoga therapy. The yoga therapy field itself is increasingly recognized as a scientifically valid approach to physical and mental health. Comprehensive Yoga Therapy is derived from classical yoga and is accessible to all people, no matter their age, weight, or abilities. Comprehensive Yoga Therapy seeks to identify your areas of imbalance. It is a beneficial therapy for people from all walks of life because it is designed to help you practice the kind of self-reflection that motivates true, lasting change in life. Based on the timeless principles of classical yoga, Comprehensive Yoga Therapy has a wealth of tools to support you in restoring life's balance.

Yoga postures are an aspect of this form of therapy; still, the real power comes from harnessing the mind/feelings and intellect to effect change on a deeper level. Many of the practices in this book tap into the roots of your stress and anxiety to transform them where they began, deep within your consciousness.

A fundamental precept is that "healing begins in the mind." In most modern cultures, yoga is defined by the standard of an exercise class: a sequence of postures, breathing exercises, some relaxation, and perhaps meditation. According to its roots, however, the word "yoga" means uniting all parts of one's life to a higher self. Therefore, the process of Comprehensive Yoga Therapy for anxiety looks at every facet of your life. This creates a synergistic effect where the sum results are more powerful than the small changes made. Throughout this book you learn specific tools to master your daily life and connect to your higher self, then your anxiety lessens as your larger understanding of things becomes clear. Your anxiety is replaced with your own confidence that your life has deep meaning.

Comprehensive Yoga Therapy applies the self-realization practices of yoga to daily life. Ancient healing methods are based on creating balance. These widespread lifestyle factors include practices for relationships, attitudes toward work, relaxation, meditation, and personally meaningful spiritual aspects, as appropriate for the clients' personal belief systems. Traditional yoga and the comprehensive lifestyle approach offer methods to alleviate suffering in the quest for harmony of body, life energy/breath, mind/feelings, intellect, and spirit/higher self. Nowadays we do a yoga class alongside other people, but a personalized yoga plan for health has to be unique and incorporate not just postures but breathing exercises, relaxation, and most importantly the power of the mind. And that's what this book provides!

The majority of people in modern society are healthy, but stress will slowly lead to imbalances in health. Healthy but stressed people are the least motivated to care for their health because they experience no pain or manifested disease condition. Comprehensive Yoga Therapy offers a structure for preventative health care in the "three Ps": Proactive, Participatory, and Personalized.

The Three Ps of Comprehensive Yoga Therapy	
Proactive	Be empowered to take control of the lifestyle factors that predispose you to ailments
Participatory	Be engaged in effecting positive change in all areas of your life
Personalized	Be viewed as an individual and receive personally meaningful tools designed to support your physical, energetic, mental, intellectual, and spiritual health

A beginner in yoga may complete all the exercises in this book; it is designed for you! Remember to practice the yoga postures in a comfortable way, so that there is never pain. If you are familiar with yoga postures, you may notice that some of the names do not match the ones you are familiar with from class. Different styles of yoga have different names for the same posture, or the same names for different postures. After developing a tradition for thousands of years, you can imagine how some discrepancies may arise; hold these lightly.

You do not need a yoga therapist to work through this book, which was written for the average reader to gain great benefit. That said, this book is not meant to replace medical or professional psychological advice. Continue working with your care providers and seek help as it would benefit you. If you have chronic depression, anxiety, or physical health issues please be sure to consult with professionals. Should you wish to connect with a Comprehensive Yoga Therapist, consult Appendix C at the end of this book.

Stress and Anxiety

You will notice in this book that for the sake of brevity, we often use the words "stress" and "anxiety" interchangeably. From a psychiatric perspective they are not the same. Where stress is typically a passing response to external influences, anxiety is a more consistent state of heightened stress. The main symptom of anxiety is exaggerated worry or tension, where people often expect the worst to happen. People also attach their anxiety to things that haven't happened yet: potential situations, losses, or emotions. Anxiety traps us in a dystopian future and disconnects us from the joy and possibility of the present moment, our current lives, and our inner resources. Anxiety is categorized in *The Diagnostic and Statistical Manual of Mental Disorders* and people are given medication to cope with it.

Both stress and anxiety activate our autonomic nervous system and create a climate of fear and doubt within us. It is these physiological, emotional, and psychological responses that we work with in this book. By learning to relax your body, master your mind, and harness your intellect to shift your thinking patterns, you can alleviate stress *and* anxiety.

How to Use This Book

Comprehensive Yoga Therapy not only pinpoints the areas of imbalance but also applies yoga philosophy and techniques to create sustained and progressive improvement in all areas of your life. Throughout this book we offer exercises to help rebalance your life for the purpose of removing stress and anxiety. These exercises were designed to help you see your life clearly, shift your thinking, and understand what powerful action steps you can take to begin improving your life right away. You don't have to do all of the exercises in the book; however, to read the book and not do the exercises could be likened to prepping a delicious meal and not cooking it. (Living a life without stress is, of course, like enjoying that scrumptious meal!)

Do not assume all the exercises in the book will benefit you equally or that they will all apply to everyone who reads the book. You are welcome to personalize your journey through this book. We designed the book with a myriad of exercises so that you can choose the ones that are most beneficial at any given time. Be sure that when you complete the exercises you honestly state how your life is now, not how you want it to be or how it used to be. This gives you a realistic starting point and helps clarify the next step. Be willing to admit that some aspects of your worldview contribute to stress and be willing to live stress-free! We suggest that you revisit this book time and again throughout your life—as you deepen and change, so will the benefits you receive from the exercises!

Although we were careful to organize the book in a systematic way, you need not read it in order. If you already feel strong in an area that we are discussing, you may choose to skip it and go to the content and exercises that address your personal areas of need. You can always come back and read over the places you missed as your self-understanding deepens and you crave more information. If an exercise in the book seems too complex, leave it and attend to the ones you are ready to work with or value.

It is okay to jump around in the book. You may discover that you are weaker in one area of your lifestyle than another. Some people have more stress at work and others at home. Some may need more relaxation practice and others more movement. The truth is, it is near impossible for one person to have an absolute life balance at one time. The magic of Comprehensive Yoga Therapy is how it balances all parts of you while strengthening the weakest link. In this book you will receive support to firmly understand and transform your life stress and anxiety. If your breathing practice falters once your relationship improves or if you stop exercising just because you balanced your work stress, you create new weak links and become vulnerable to stress. Thus, this book supports you in honing your healthy lifestyle in all areas while removing stress and anxiety; you decide which order is best.

We suggest you get a journal of some kind for working through this book. You can have fun with this and select a notebook with an inspiring cover that helps you feel happy, strong, and alive when you look at it. Some people also get a special pen to make writing in the journal more enticing. You can use this journal not only for completing the exercises of this book but also to vent your frustrations, share your dreams, work through problems, clarify confusion, congratulate yourself, or track your goals such as yoga home practice, nutrition, or emotional balance.

Stay connected to your deep motivation. If you follow this book and start to feel better, do your very best to stick with the practices! If you discontinue living the lessons from this book, that insidious anxiety may return. People will notoriously pay far more money and take greater action to avoid pain than seek pleasure because pain is a terrific motivator! People act with great dedication to remove pain but as soon as it goes away, so does the effort to maintain the helpful behaviors and inevitably a slide occurs. This book teaches you a deeper motivation so that you are not so pain-focused. This book reminds you that it is possible to remove stress from a person. Notice that I said "remove stress from a *person*," not "remove stress from life." Stress—illness, lists, deadlines, mistakes, and the like—will come into everyone's life. It has throughout human existence. Removing stress is not about waiting for external circumstances to change, which keeps us stressed. Instead, we turn inward and take ownership over the beliefs that created stress and anxiety in the first place. Although stress is a part of life, this book helps you understand what creates a stress-filled life and what builds a life of ease instead. Feeling good keeps you motivated.

You will gain new insights throughout this book as we use some of the tools offered by the tradition of yoga. In Part I we will use basic tools of science, physiology, and psychology to soothe anxiety, including the ancient concept of the layers of a human being (*koshas*). In Part II we guide you along the five paths of yoga: psychology (*raja*), intellect (*jnana*), mind-body health (*tantra*), work (*karma*), and relationships (*bhakti*). Part III gives you the tools to work through your resistances to well-being and offers practical techniques to support your growth in the direction of freedom and ease. Each chapter includes some elements of yoga philosophy, breathing, postures, meditation, nutrition, relaxation/sleep, and personal attitudes. There is a point-form summary at the end of each chapter to help you retain the salient points and quickly review the material.

You will notice italicized words in parentheses throughout the book. These words are from the tradition of yoga, in the ancient language of Sanskrit. There are no direct translations for these words; however, we have included a glossary to begin to define them for you. If you choose to deepen your study of yoga, broadening your understanding of these concepts may be important. For now, have the benefit of how these concepts support you in balancing your life and removing stress and anxiety.

Yoga Therapy for Stress and Anxiety: The Process

This is a transformative step-by-step process. As you work through this book you will be guided by your own, personally meaningful intention that you will create in Chapter 1. Through the perspectives and practices outlined throughout the book, you will reprogram your nervous system to dial back the fight-flight-or-freeze mode and dial up the rest-and-digest mode. Gradually, you will feel more confident in challenging the beliefs and nonconscious thought patterns that perpetuate anxiety. As you work through this book, you will address each of the main areas of life affected by anxiety, becoming clearer about your own areas of weakness and strength. The science of modern psychology directly relates to many fundamental yoga concepts. Yoga's ancient philosophies and techniques are sometimes repackaged for a modern world, but their roots and outcomes are the same. This book applies yoga philosophy, breathing, postures, meditation, nutrition, relaxation/sleep, and personal attitudes to removing stress and anxiety.

It's in your power to decide how you want your life to be. We wrote this book to put you back in control of your life and it is important for you to remember that you truly are the one in control. That doesn't mean it will feel true all the time; however, as you follow the exercises and information outlined here, you will come to see how much potential there is for you to gain complete mastery over your life and claim your right to peace. You will likely focus on the chapters that most relate to your disposition. For example, the career-oriented will follow Chapter 8, the scholar may be drawn to Chapter 6, the emotional person Chapter 9, the worrier Chapter 3, and so on. Different people are more strongly active through different filters, and this can change through the course of life. Those who focus on Chapter 7, for example, likely filter through the body and Chapter 5 through the psyche. Follow your frame of reference while at the same time considering points of view from the other paths and how they can help free you from stress and anxiety.

How This Book Came About

The impetus of this book was that, as yoga therapists and Comprehensive Yoga Therapy Trainers, we have seen an epidemic of stress in our society. We have also seen the benefit that yoga classes and yoga therapy have brought to countless people on their journeys out of stress and anxiety. Below, each of us shares our own journey into this project.

Bob: My search for meaning in life began before the word "stress" was popular. As a college student, I was experiencing a persistent confusion related to making the right choices for my future life: I was torn between the lofty goal of working toward world peace via political channels and interpersonal channels. The indecisiveness about how to use my life as a tool to alleviate as much suffering in the world as possible, ironically, began causing me suffering.

As I progressed positively in this spiritual path, one of my closest mentors in Japan adamantly recommended that I take the six-month onsite yoga teacher's training course at The Yoga Institute in Mumbai, so long as I was able to receive the advanced training, which included individual mentorship. Miraculously, this occurred and I met with Dr. Jayadeva Yogendra and Hansaji Yogendra on a daily basis for one hour of private study in the midst of the daily yoga therapist training at the residential school. Being at one of the first-ever locations to apply yoga as a therapy for health conditions, I was introduced to the approach that you will find in this book. The ancient science of yoga has examined every aspect of human life from the physical seen in the yoga posture practices to the mental, psychological, and spiritual. The yoga lifestyle elements that relate to relationships, work, and nutrition are also key aspects to the healthy living program at The Yoga Institute. The Comprehensive Yoga Therapy program is formally recognized by The Yoga Institute as carrying forward this tradition that applies the ancient teachings of yoga to help with one of humanity's major problems: stress. Enjoy this book that applies a harmonious team of authors to communicate the clearest book possible. Blessings to your life journey!

Erin: I believe in yoga so much that it has been my life's work. Yoga therapy for post-traumatic stress was the topic of my graduate thesis in counseling psychology. Bob and I met through a mutual friend, and with his PhD in yoga therapy, he served as my academic mentor during that time. Over the ten years of being a psychotherapist, I worked with a lot of people suffering from anxiety. I have been teaching yoga for many years and almost every student begins classes saying they are looking for something to help with their stress. Yoga does that! When Bob and I collaborated to create Comprehensive Yoga Therapist Training, we were mindful of addressing anxiety and stress in a positive, therapeutic, and empowering way. It has been a joy to share the endeavor of this book with my esteemed CYTT colleagues and friends Bob and Staffan. I had terrific fun inventing some of the exercises in this book, sharing stories from our community, and giving my voice to this work. It is my sincere hope that you benefit from these efforts and live into the freedom, ease, and peace that is yours to claim!

Staffan: I graduated from physical therapy school in 1985. I got a great education in anatomy, exercise, and manual skills. My education served me well and I was supporting the high-level athletes that I had always dreamed of working with. After practicing for a few years, I came to the realization that many of my clients were not responding as well as I had hoped for. I, and the health care field as a whole, was missing something. I studied the Feldenkrais Method for four years and studied meditation with Thich Nhat Hanh. I felt as if I was getting closer, but I was still missing something. I started studying yoga at YogaLife in Devon, Pennsylvania. Those studies combined with my background in the Feldenkrais Method and physical therapy led me to where I am now. The additional benefits of the Comprehensive Yoga Therapy approach are obvious to both my clients and me. While writing this book it has also become clear to me that science is catching up with yoga and other mindfulness approaches. Thanks to new noninvasive imaging techniques we can now look at how the structure of the brain changes with stress and how it changes when we practice mindfulness. The changes are more rapid than previously thought. I have truly enjoyed adding to the anatomy and science sections of this book, and I know that the reader will benefit from the Comprehensive Yoga Therapy approach as a way to reduce stress and anxiety.

This yoga therapy book is based on yoga teachings and techniques that have been recommended for generations. Although society has changed, these ancient approaches to well-being remain potent and effective. May you be enriched by your insights while reading and reflecting on the exercises that follow. Going through this process requires you to be patient with yourself: keep the faith and have some fun!

Part I: Foundations of Stress and Anxiety

In Part I of this book, we will introduce the main habits that keep us feeling stressed and exacerbate anxiety. First, we explain stress and anxiety and how yoga therapy helps those conditions. We discuss mental habits and beliefs that interrupt your peace of mind and offer exercises that help connect to a sense of greater self-understanding, confidence, and ease. We talk about the relationship between body, breath, mind/feelings, intellect, and spirit/higher self. Yoga theory and practice are interwoven through the chapters to give you a direct experience of the topics.

Chapter 1

Yoga Therapy's Role in Relieving Stress and Anxiety

This chapter relates stressful experiences to your biology, physiology, and lifestyle. We begin by describing stress and anxiety in the modern context. The exercises and ideas in this chapter give you a solid foundation for building an anxiety-free life through the rest of the book.

Anxiety Lifestyle

Most people's lives are set up to keep them anxious. Unreasonable work demands, strained relationships, violent news reports, and frustrating traffic are just a few of the everyday worries most people face. Approximately 15 percent of people will experience a diagnosed anxiety disorder in their lives, with hundreds of millions of dollars being spent on anti-anxiety medication every year. With more than forty million clinically anxious people in the United States alone, it is easy to see that we are living in a culture where worry is out of hand. The people in these statistics typically have their basic needs for food and shelter met. Many of them have everything they could hope for on the surface, with healthy families and stable jobs and good friends. However, on the inside there remains a sense of fear, worry, or dissatisfaction. There is an emotional knowing that says something is missing or could go wrong. In this absence of faith, anxiety arises. Even though our water is potable, we are perpetually entertained, and we can communicate at the click of a button, something feels amiss.

Technology has advanced, leading us to spend more time on our own indoors without deep relationships, including a connection to ourselves. While technological development has increased rapidly over the last few decades, yoga class size has also been increasing. Every day we see more people looking for a permanent way to rid themselves of stress—people who have been suffering from anxiety, many of whom are in the care of a physician. Despite this, the anxiety continues and people seek other paths to freedom.

Longtime yoga students live the example of contentment and when their stressed-out friends ask why they've been so relaxed the last few years they tell them, "It's the yoga." That's not to say that doing a few stretches makes stress go away. However, in a culture that promotes stress through its pace and value systems, it's beneficial to experience time dedicated to going inward. Within us resides a well of deep and abiding peace—the higher self. Although this confident, peaceful well is easily covered by lists, emails, and traffic, the higher self is always there, waiting for us to connect.

As people seek a way out of anxiety, and stronger skills to cope with stress, they turn to yoga more and more as a means of quieting the inner turmoil. Yoga philosophy and practices are designed to calm and quiet us. Originally conceived by sages as a path to enlightenment, yoga methods systematically move us in the direction of deep, peaceful understanding and freedom from worry. The ethical principles, movements, breathing practices, and mind-quieting techniques—all of which you will experience via the exercises of this book—unwind stressful habits and carve a path to a wellspring of confident well-being within your higher self.

Throughout this book we offer you recommendations and suggestions to connect to who you really are—your higher self. You are embarking upon a spiritual journey of transcending stress and anxiety and moving into confidence and ease. Let's play a language game to get a feel for the underlying process of transforming stress and anxiety into personal confidence and ease. The English word "confidence" is made up of two Latin words:

Con = together
Fido = with trust

Trust, or faith, is required in order for us to feel strong, capable, and relaxed; thus, there is a spiritual component to removing stress and anxiety.

"Ease" comes from the Old French for comfort, pleasure, well-being, or opportunity. Reread each of those four defining words and notice the effect they have on your body, breath, and state of mind. Do you feel a little safer or calmer? The old definition of ease also has to do with a sense of physical rest, which relates to the role of yoga postures in freeing us from stress.

The word "stress" actually means "narrowness" or "oppression." How trapped or tightly wound we feel when under stress! "Anxiety" is from the Latin for "to choke." Yikes!

Stress that leads to anxiety = absence of confidence

When we feel stressed, we are lacking trust, faith, confidence, ease, and peace of mind. Peace comes from a confidence in our ability to connect with the higher self and handle situations with self-reliance. With a sense of confidence and personal mastery over your inner world, you will come together with your higher self, in trust. Once we understand that the higher self is always present, we can shift our thinking and act with courage and ease. Consequently, as yoga therapy practices establish us in the experience of the higher self, we are motivated to take action to change anything that disturbs our minds.

How Comprehensive Yoga Therapy Works

Comprehensive Yoga Therapy addresses the needs of the body, life energy, emotions, thoughts, and spirit/higher self. On the spiritual level, the realm of the higher self, we already possess everything we need. These resources may be untapped, but this book gives you the tools to connect with them! Solutions to your problems will surface as you practice the exercises in this book. You will experience yogic techniques of witnessing your thoughts and feelings and quieting emotions. Deep breathing steadies your mind, soothes emotions, and relaxes your body. Targeted relaxations use the power of the mind to soften rigid muscles and calm the nervous and endocrine systems. Yoga postures uplift emotions while strengthening and steadying the body-mind complex. These basic tools presented in this book are readily available to you and can be immediately applied—most of them anytime and anywhere!

We are embarking upon a journey together with this book. Trust the process of removing stress. Gradually, as you observe yourself and apply the teachings and exercises from this book, you will see yourself begin to respond differently to problems. Little things that used to upset you will become less painful; you will no longer be annoyed by things out of your control. Does this take time? Sure, but with only a little practice you will notice that you are different. Let this encourage you! Appreciate the small victories, knowing they are signs of all the goodness to come as you read the book, practice the exercises, and commit yourself to a life without anxiety.

Lifestyle changes become more and more important in today's society, where our routines tend to be colored by unhealthy activities. Yoga therapy can make the biggest impact by guiding people through simple, powerful shifts in daily routines. Thinking back over the last couple of centuries, people did not talk about stress as a pervasive problem the way they do today. Although there have always been pains and problems in life, in times gone by there was more space for the mind to work them out. Think of how beneficial a short walk, chat with a friend, or healthy meal is to your stress. Historically, walking was the mainstay of travel, communities of families and neighbors visited almost nightly, and food was grown and cooked by the same people eating it. A traditional lifestyle was full of hard work, but the benefits were celebrated. We fill our modern lives with electronic interactions and information, rarely giving the mind or nervous system a chance to rest, process, or truly connect with others.

Today there are so many options to choose from when it comes to how to make a living. In traditional societies you did what your family did, or what the tribe decided that they needed, or what your calling was determined to be. These days, a student starts college with a major in mind, but after a while may doubt that choice and get confused by all the options. If you are not successful, or even if you are, you may very well be anxious about whether or not you made the right decision in life.

Many people are on medication because of their stress and anxiety. *The Diagnostic and Statistical Manual of Mental Disorders*, now in its fifth edition (DSM-5), is a psychiatric tool used to classify, label, and diagnose disorders. Once a label is applied, it helps define which course of medication and treatment is appropriate. The DSM-5 says that there are many forms of anxiety. Issues falling under the classification of anxiety disorders include (but are not limited to) acute stress disorder, panic disorder, specific phobias, obsessive-compulsive disorder, post-traumatic stress disorder, and generalized anxiety disorder. Other psychiatric disorders with overlapping symptoms include categories of mood, dissociative, somatoform, eating, sleep, sexual, autism, and adjustment disorders. The diagnostic label serves to offer a medicalized path of treatment. While you may not "meet the diagnostic criteria" of a certain anxiety disorder, stress can bring great detriment to your life. Yoga therapy seeks to move in the direction of health, without diagnosis, and works with shifting the behaviors and beliefs related to anxiety. By altering daily routines, your entire approach to life can be transformed. This works because the shape of life is different, but it also has biological effects!

Your brain is three brains in one, and all three brains relate to your stress and anxiety. The hindbrain is common to all vertebrates. It is colloquially called the reptilian brain and is responsible for ensuring our instinctual needs—breathing, eating, drinking, and resting—are met. This brain keeps us in survival mode and it rules us when we feel unsafe. The mammalian brain, or limbic system, wraps around the reptilian brain and is common to all our warm-blooded kin. It relates to our basic emotional needs, such as touch, community, language, reproduction, and play. The neocortex, which wraps around the mammalian brain, is unique to humans and other higher primates. This human brain is associated with higher reason, forethought, and the ability to attribute meaning to experiences. It is not fully developed until our mid-twenties! Each of these brains relates to how and why we experience stress.

In order to balance our lifestyle, we must consider these three brains. The foundation of a stress-free life is to keep that reptilian part of ourselves content. Eat nutritious food according to the body's satiety cues and stay hydrated. Rest enough. It is key in activating the body's healing resources, remaining relaxed, and integrating emotional experiences. While sex is a basic bodily need, we can meet this through other physical and creative activities as well by calling upon the higher mind. We are pack animals; connection and play are essential to our well-being. Children who are not touched enough do not thrive. People who laugh more are generally healthier. Throughout history games have shaped our culture and helped us blow off steam. Socializing more benefits this animalistic part of our nature. We nourish the human brain by continuing to learn and grow, seeking and inserting personal meaning into everyday existence through spiritual connection. We change over time, hopefully moving in the direction of alignment with who we truly are and the vision of that peaceful, contented higher self.

Where are You?

Maybe your life is starting to get stressful. Perhaps you have been struggling with anxiety for some time. Let's take a deep breath before we evaluate where you are with your anxiety at this time. ... There, that's better. The most common benefit from our yoga classes is deep breathing because it nourishes the entire body as well as eases emotions and slows the thoughts. You will get the most out of reading this book in a relaxed state. We wish to ensure that every time you pick up this book you check that your breath is deep, slow, and steady. You may even bring a slight smile to your face so that the reading and self-reflection experience is joyful, peaceful, and healing.

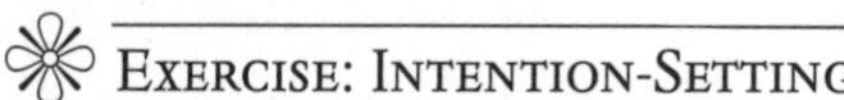

Exercise: Intention-Setting

All of us wish our lives could be free from stress. Yoga doesn't distinguish between the different sources of stress; it acknowledges that stress is a state that separates us from the higher self. Stress may come from a spinal injury, a loved one passing, or problems with coworkers, and freedom from stress comes from self-awareness. Whatever may be the source of your stress or anxiety, yoga is a path to freedom. Use this exercise to help clarify your path out of stress and anxiety. It is important to understand the meaning behind your endeavor. Your personal intention will support and inspire you throughout this process. Throughout your healing journey with this book, write down your feelings and insights. You may get a special journal for these thoughts and to complete the exercises you will do through this course. You may revisit this exercise many times as you read through this book. It is normal for your intention to shift, evolve, or refine as you work through the exercises and gain greater self-understanding. Allow your intention to keep you focused on your journey out of stress and anxiety.

1. Ask yourself: "Why did I open this book?" The answer is not as simple as saying you don't want stress anymore. You have a specific, personal reason why you don't want it. Write that reason down. To help clarify, you may reflect or journal on the following questions in order to refine your intention.
    - Why are you reading this book?
    - What do you want to learn?
    - How will your life be different when you are free from anxiety?
    - What is your personal intention for reading this book?
2. To strengthen your intention, state it in the positive. Your mind will hold the words that it focuses on so it is best to intend what you want. For example, if your intention is "To not be afraid of work," then your mind reflects on "be afraid." If your intention is "To feel confident and at ease at work," your mind creates the feeling of confidence and imagines you going through your workdays with ease. Have fun creating your intention and remember this is just for you—there is no right or wrong intention!

3. If you wish to dig into your intention more deeply, you may start to ask yourself "Why?" "Why do I want to stay calm at work?" "Why am I hoping for confidence?" At first the answer seems obvious—to not feel bad anymore! If you let yourself go deeper, you may realize there are underlying reasons to your desires: "If I handle stress at work better, I will be respected more and may be able to implement some of my ideas." "If I had confidence I would do more of the things I love instead of life passing me by." Do you see how these deeper intentions are inherently more motivating and meaningful?
4. Give yourself a chance to understand the spiritual aspect of this desire. Follow the intention of your higher self. You may repeat this process of asking "why" until you connect with a virtue such as balance, faith, trust, hope, acceptance, forgiveness, patience. This isn't necessary, however; for now it is enough to have a simple idea to guide you as you practice this book.

After you define your initial intention, follow this book to continue exploring your intention. Whenever you start something new, there is a learning curve. What this means is, you won't be as skilled in the beginning as you will be after some practice. You won't get it right every time! Do not allow letdowns to undermine your intentions. Cultivating peace, ease, confidence, and freedom from anxiety is a lifelong endeavor. Do not quit just because your anxiety returns or you forget to apply practices. Trust these slips as part of the learning curve and know that you are refining yourself and your life.

Keep your intention before you and allow it to filter all of your efforts. You can avert potential disappointments by remembering your role in your own process as you progress on the path of yoga. By acting with this personal intention in view, you have a clear, internal focus to measure your efforts, rather than looking to subjective, external outcomes that are often beyond your control. Yoga is not a magic wand; the effort *you* put into it will offer results.

The Spark of Effort and Discipline (*Tapas*)

One of the main precepts of yoga is effort/discipline (*tapas*), which translates as "to generate light or heat." This refers to the psychic energy generated through consistent practice. It is important to be balanced in our efforts. Some people have a tendency to be too hard or critical in approach while others are too soft or lazy. When we try too hard, we create thought disturbances. If we do not try hard enough, we create thought disturbances. A balance between effort and detachment is key. This means patiently keeping a daily practice. Effort is a means through which we can connect to the higher self. We acknowledge the importance of discipline/effort and moderation in helping us carry out routine and our commitment to eradicating anxiety. Through establishing a daily rhythm guided by yoga, we develop a conditioned and still mind, as opposed to being stressed and unfocused. Once established in routine, it takes care of itself. It's just what we do. Remember how every day when you were a child your parents had to tell you to brush your teeth? Now, as an adult, it's just a part of your routine. Ultimately, the regularity of a daily practice saves us from pain and suffering.

Understand that effort is a powerful quality of your higher self. Painful childhood experiences may make you think of discipline as punishment, which contributes to the idle or harsh styles of motivation. As adults, it is possible to recognize discipline as a gift that helps develop confidence, ease, and inner strength. Allow your effort to be moderate and consistent over the long term, warming you and lighting your path. If you miss a day (or a week, or a year) of practicing your intention, it is okay; simply restart as soon as possible and go forward.

All of the traditional texts of yoga repeat that the way you align with your higher self is through constant practice (yes, that's *constant*), over a long period of time (this from a culture who believes in reincarnation—that is a very long time!), without attachment to the end results. Our continual effort "lights a fire" under us, offering enthusiasm and inspiration for the effort. The heat of effort stings us when we don't want to practice, and that small burn of resistance reminds us that we are purifying our lives through practice, just as fire burns impurities from gold. All the while, ironically, we are not attached to the results of our efforts. However, by following this yoga lifestyle practice, the rewards of our efforts fall into open hands. Immediate progress is evident in subtle ways, such as taking more quiet time or not being irked by small irritants. When we integrate effort into our lives, we gradually establish a routine of practice. This daily rhythm helps us restrain from impulses, regulate desires, accept internal authority, and achieve personal mastery. Put your energy toward the effort of practice and remain relaxed through the process.

Exercise: Meeting the Challenge of Change

Are you ready to transform your stress? "Yes!" Do you want to live without anxiety? "Yes!" Are you willing to change your habits? "Uhh, which habits do you want me to change? That might be too hard." It's normal for us to balk at the idea of change; in fact, yoga philosophy teaches that fear of change is one of the main obstacles to peace of mind. Some of the following questions may seem strange or counterintuitive; just do your best to answer truthfully as you experiment with your own ideas, hopes, and resistances about change. No one has to know.

1. Really ask yourself: "Why do I want to be free from anxiety?"
2. If you give up stress and anxiety, what else do you have to give up? What could you no longer do/think/say/feel/believe if you were stress-free? Do not dismiss these questions; look deeply into yourself and see if there are inklings of answers.
3. How is your life better because you are stressed? How do stress and anxiety help you in your life?
4. Will life be better if you transform your stress and anxiety? How? In what ways will you be more like your higher self?

Exercise: Bringing Intention (*Sankalpa*) to Yoga Postures

The state of your body directly relates to your state of mind. In the next two chapters you will learn more about beliefs and the mind-body complex (*chitta*). For now, notice that relaxing the body can help soothe the mind. Many of us live disconnected from our intention for doing things, whether in work, relationships, or some other area of life. By holding your intention, or by simply being aware of passing impressions during practice, notice that you found a way to strengthen your state of mind through yoga postures! As you apply your pure goals or intentions in yoga postures, you'll start to do the same in your daily actions. As you practice the following yoga postures, hold your intention in mind to amplify the benefits.

1. Before beginning the yoga postures, record the current quality of your thoughts and feelings. The following yoga postures give you a chance to practice embodying your higher self as you keep your mind focused on your intention.
2. Repeat each of these gentle yoga postures a few times, keeping your mind on your intention. You may recite it slowly, like a mantra, or call in the feeling of your intention. You may imagine yourself living that way or feel the way various postures represent your intention. Be creative and have fun exploring how you can relate your intention to yoga postures. Begin with the first posture, completing it a comfortable number of times (two to ten times is fine) before moving on to the next posture. Be sure to complete the entire sequence in order to enjoy an anatomically balanced practice. If you don't have much time, it is okay to do each pose once. Move slowly with each deep inhale and exhale, feeling activation in your body but no pain.

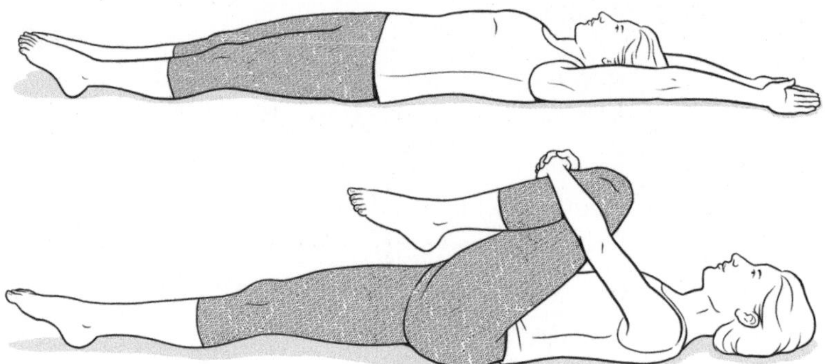

Figures 1.1a and 1.1b
a. Yastikasana/Pavana Muktasana (Stick Pose/Wind-Releasing Pose)

Lying on your back, inhale both arms overhead, placing the back of your hands on the floor over your head. Stretch from the waist and middle back in either direction to make your body as long as possible while keeping your shoulders relaxed (*Yastikasana*). Exhale and draw the right knee toward the chest, holding gently with both hands either at the shin or behind the knee. You may flex your toes toward the sky (*Pavana Muktasana*). Repeat the inhale, stretching your body long, and open into *Yastikasana*. Exhale the other (left) knee to the chest, holding with both hands while the heels press outward and toes reach up. This posture offers a full body stretch and may be practiced independently of other poses. For those of you whose stress affects digestion, there is the added benefit of activating peristalsis and elimination.

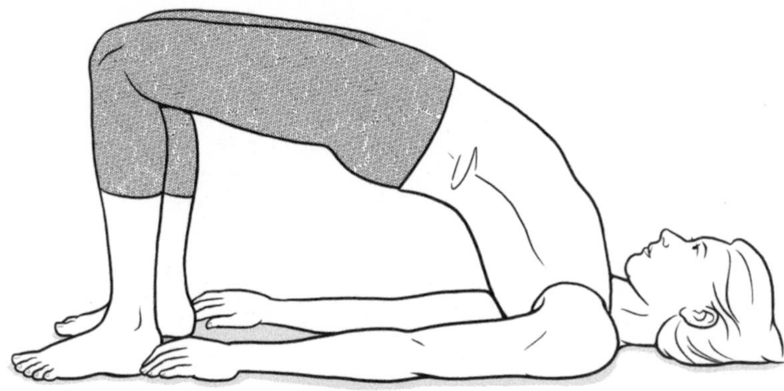

Figure 1.2
b. Setu Bandhasana **(Bridge Pose)**

Rest on your back and bend your knees, bringing them hip-width apart with feet planted close to buttocks. Ensure feet and knees remain in line with the hips through the entire pose rather than collapsing them in or out. Inhale and roll the pelvis and lower back upward from the mat. Continue breathing deeply, feeling your ribs expand to the sides and back of your body. Hold for a comfortable time, breathing regularly and grounding into your legs and feet before lowering on an exhale with slow control. This posture helps deepen the breath and connect you to the ground for a feeling of safety.

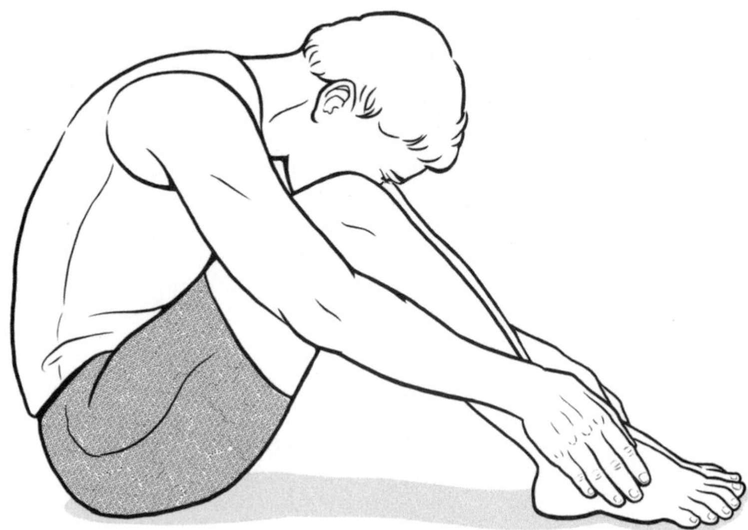

Figure 1.3
c. Restorative Forward Bend

Come to a seated position. Soles of the feet on the floor, similar to the posture above, exhale and rest the front of your body on your thighs, resting your forehead on your knees. You may need to fold your arms on the knees to create a pillow for your head; otherwise, rest them alongside the legs. Feel your entire body relaxing with each exhale. Hold for roughly ten breaths to give the muscles and mind sufficient time to relax, then roll up gently, with the help of your arms.

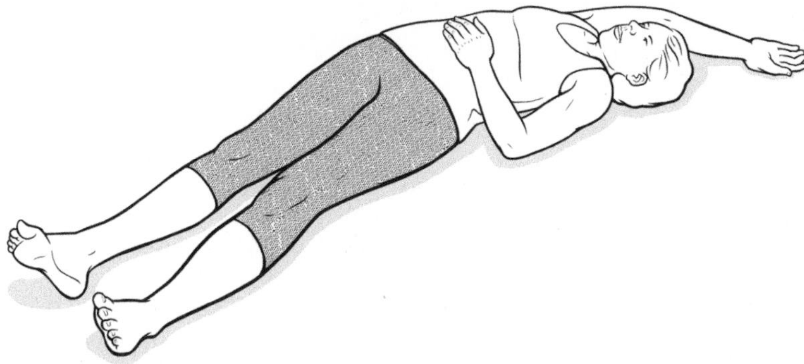

Figure 1.4
d. *Supta Ardha Chandrasana* **(Supine Half-Moon Pose)**

Straighten your legs out along the floor and walk your feet to the left side, resting your left hand on your abdomen. If appropriate, raise your right arm alongside your ear, back of hand resting on the floor (bend the elbow if necessary). Notice your breath in the right side of your body. Repeat on the other side, knowing this posture is cleansing and supportive.

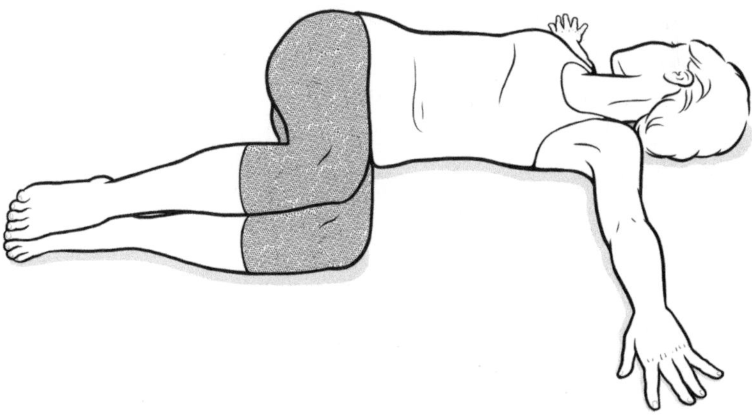

Figure 1.5
e. *Supta Matsyendrasana* **(Reclined Half Twist)**

Extend your arms to the sides in a "T" position at shoulder height and bring your knees to your chest. To protect your back, keep your feet on the floor at all times; otherwise, your knees can go right into your chest. Exhale your legs to one side and ensure that your feet are supported by the earth. If you are free from neck issues, turn your face gently in the opposite direction of your knees. With practice, your thighs may come to a right angle to your torso and both shoulders may rest on the floor. Surrender into the support of the ground. Postures like this one that revolve the spine increase circulation there and help regulate the nervous system, thereby soothing any undue anxiety. Relax your forehead and abdomen to amplify this effect. Repeat the posture on the other side.

3. After relaxing on your back or belly for a few breaths, notice the effect of intention, breath, and yoga postures on your thoughts, emotions, and sense of connection to who you really are, your higher self. Notice the current quality of your thoughts and feelings. Journal your observations, then compare them to what you wrote in Step 1 of this exercise, before you did the yoga posture practice. How did these simple movements impact your internal sense of relaxation, ease, and connection to your higher self?

Exercise: Morning Breath

What difference would it make in your life if every morning began with calming connection? This exercise offers you a simple practice that can be done daily in very little time for big impact on easing stress and anxiety!

1. Begin each day with three deep breaths, thinking of your current spiritual intention. (Note: Laughter works as an alternative to deep breaths!)
2. The closer to awakening that you perform this exercise, the more effective it will be. This practice sets the tone for the day, shifting consciousness to a calm perspective before you face any challenges. It has the additional bonus of low-

ering your nervous system's baseline of stress, relaxing you even more before the day gets going so when stresses occur, you can slough them off more easily. This helps inoculate you against the cumulative effects of stress throughout the day. You can return to a conscious intention via deep breath whenever you choose!

Exercise: Taoist Smile

Have you ever rushed through a store, harried, frustrated, pressed for time, and had a stranger smile at you? Immediately, the connection is soothing. How about the experience of being alone in your car, sad and stressed, and pulling up beside someone at a red light who is grinning or singing loudly? It can instantly shift your tone. A smile is a force to be reckoned with. The ancient Taoists knew this and taught the self-care technique of the inner smile.

1. Begin forming a smile, gradually widening it to a huge grin. It's okay if you don't feel like grinning, just put your facial muscles into that happy-looking posture.
2. Notice the feeling of your smiling muscles: the upward tug of your lips, the squint of your eyes, the relaxed forehead. You may notice the smile brings other sensations throughout your body, as well.
3. Feel the presence of the smile in your mind, perhaps in the form of happy images, uplifting emotions, or a general calm. Feel your body light up, as if showered by smiles.
4. Let the grin soften, leaving a peaceful upward curve of your lips, and mentally move the soft smile to your forehead, releasing any lingering thoughts.
5. Feel the smile permeate your skull, then cascade down your neck and shoulders, filling toward your torso.
6. Move the smile into your heart and create a peaceful acceptance of any emotions that may reside there. There is no

need to avoid or resist, simply feel the emotions with a peaceful awareness.

7. Allow the smile to continue through your body, resting in the stomach region, relaxing the diaphragm. Feel it flow through your guts and down your spine, drifting down your legs to your feet.
8. Bask in the smiling feeling shining through your entire body. This simple practice can be applied at any time to feed yourself contentment. When happiness is present, fear cannot exist. When we smile, we cannot feel nervous. When we feel good, we start smiling. Our facial muscles are engaged in a certain pattern. The brain recognizes this pattern and releases endorphins and dopamine. We feel joyful. More than likely we can use the same feedback loop in reverse: that is, we smile to feel good. The brain will recognize the pattern of muscle activation and release feel-good neurotransmitters. It takes practice, though. Babies are said to smile hundreds of times a day. Adults smile forty to fifty times and sometimes not even that many. Maybe if we "forced" ourselves to smile as frequently as a baby we would automatically be happier and less anxious. Enjoy the experience of the smile uplifting your sense of physical, emotional, and mental well-being.

Anxiety is Literally a "Nervous Condition"

The autonomic nervous system (ANS) in our bodies consists of the sympathetic (SNS) and parapsympathetic (PNS) branches. The SNS is activated during stressful situations that lead to the fight-flight-or-freeze syndrome. The heart rate and blood pressure increase, more blood goes out to the muscles and less to the digestive system. The whole system goes on high alert, prepared to do whatever is necessary to save itself—fight or flee—or becomes paralyzed from fear. When the stress passes, the fight-flight-or-freeze activation of the SNS decreases and the PNS is activated. This rest-and-digest mode of functioning allows physical healing and rest from the high-alert stress state. At least, that is how it should work.

In today's society many people are driven by a constant activation of the SNS. It might be stress at work, at home, in relationships, or monetary stress that drives the SNS response. Constant low-level stress that is not really a "true" fight-flight-or-freeze situation can also lead to constant inhibition of the PNS, which means that the body-mind complex rarely or never finds a rest-and-digest state. In addition, worries about the future can activate the SNS and lead to inhibition of the PNS. The ANS does not know the difference between real and imagined fight-or-flight situations! For many of us, fight-or-flight is not available, so instead the third "F" (freeze) is our response. Freeze also activates the SNS, since it is a response to real or imagined danger, and organizes the body in a protective posture, which also feeds into SNS activation.

We can say that anxiety is a brain/whole body pattern disorder. Comprehensive Yoga Therapy techniques affect both branches of the ANS, and can change the mental and physical patterns that we habitually embody when we encounter stress. Yoga techniques are well known to affect the ANS and each branch, as well as shifting thoughts and physical reactions to stress. By using the yoga therapy techniques described in this book, you can discover your own patterns that lead to anxiety and then change those patterns.

As well as increasing heart rate, blood pressure, and frequency of breathing, activation of the SNS also decreases our ability to absorb nutrients and puts the body and all its organs on high alert. The SNS is a system that uses a lot of energy and does not allow the body to rest, heal, integrate emotions and experiences, or repair itself. The PNS, on the other hand, calms the body. When the PNS is activated it slows down the heart rate, decreases blood pressure, allows regular digestion, and the whole body can go into a state of rest and healing.

Our breathing is influenced by the activation of the sympathetic and parasympathetic nervous systems, but the reverse is also true. That is, the SNS and PNS are influenced by our breathing. When we pay attention to our breath, especially the exhalation phase, and utilize the diaphragmatic, slow breathing techniques suggested in the exercises below, we can activate the parasympathetic nervous system and allow our bodies to shift into a restful state of healing.

Exercise: The Diaphragmatic (Belly) Breath

Diaphragmatic, or belly, breathing ensures that the major muscle associated with healthy breathing (the diaphragm) is mobilized. The diaphragm is the muscle that lies below the lungs and plays a major role in breathing. The diaphragmatic breath is important for staying relaxed because the majority of the lungs' blood flow, and therefore gas exchange, is concentrated in the lowest lobes of the lungs. This increased oxygen absorption leads to a strong, steady mind and increased vitality as the PNS is activated. It is imperative to learn awareness and control of this essential muscle in order to maximize the potential of your breath. The movement of the belly helps circulate blood, which is relaxing to the heart. This type of breath is also recommended for emotional control—especially anxiety—because it gives you the time and space to become quiet, increasing internal awareness and emotional integration.

1. To make it as soothing as possible in the beginning, practice this exercise lying comfortably on your back and pull your knees up, placing your feet on the floor and tenting your knees together. Place one hand on your belly and one on your chest.
2. Feel the belly rise and fall into your hand as your breath flows in and out. Contract the muscles of your belly as you exhale and allow the belly to rise as you inhale. Monitor your chest using your other hand, as there will more than likely be some movement in the chest with your breathing. Don't strain to stop your chest from expanding with the in breath. Just observe what happens and see if you can focus on the movement of your belly. People with a lot of stress sometimes reverse the contraction and expansion; remember that as the lungs expand like balloons, the belly will rise and as the lungs deflate, the belly will come back down. Keep your abdomen relaxed and do not force the breath.
3. Bring a slight smile to your face as you steady the rhythm of your breath, starting with a 3-second count in and a 3-second count out. You may increase the count as comfortable to a maximum

of 10 seconds in and out. Perform ten rounds, where one inhale and exhale cycle is considered a round.

4. Feel the effects on your nervous system. Do you notice warmth, tingling, relaxation? Do you feel a sense of alertness, calm, confidence, or ease? No need to judge; simply observe and acknowledge. Record your observations in your journal.

You may choose to practice this exercise regularly. You will likely notice different effects on different days and can actually use the diaphragmatic breath as a gauge of your well-being.

Chapter Summary

1. Going through this book is a process. Trust yourself and stay connected.
2. Breathe from the diaphragm with a slight smile on your face.
3. Believe that anxiety is temporary and not an aspect of who you are.
4. Accept where you are at this time in life, knowing it will continually change.
5. The path of yoga is for life, not just until anxiety (or whatever you are working on) dissipates.
6. Stress transformation and freedom from anxiety begin and end with your intention.
7. Remember that stress is a condition of your nervous system, exacerbated by your thoughts, beliefs, and physical tensions. Relaxation is also cultivated through the nervous system.
8. A healthy lifestyle choice must be coupled with internal motivation and peace in order to be truly healthy.
9. Confidence arises from faith in yourself and in life, and helps you remain peaceful.
10. In order to balance your lifestyle, you must consider the three brains: reptilian, by meeting your biological needs; mammalian,

by meeting your social needs; and human, by meeting your spiritual needs.

11. Take a few deep breaths first thing every day.
12. Feed yourself contentment, ease, and peace through the Taoist Smile.
13. Modern gadgets and lifestyle rarely give the mind or nervous system a chance to rest, process, or truly connect with others.
14. Fear of change, one of the main afflictions of the mind, is balanced by effort/discipline. In yoga terms this translates as "generate light or heat," which can refer to "lighting a fire" under yourself, "the burn" of resistance, and the pure psychic energy of consistent practice.
15. Pure effort, versus lazy or critical disciplines, ultimately develops other virtues such as peacefulness, compassion, and confidence.
16. Balance effort of practice with detachment to the end results and gradually establish a routine.
17. Yoga therapy can make the biggest impact by guiding people through simple, powerful lifestyle changes moving in the direction of health by shifting the behaviors and beliefs related to anxiety. You increase awareness, build on healthy habits, and remove ineffective behaviors and thought patterns. Yoga therapy, without labeling or diagnosis, is truly beneficial in working with "chronic lifestyle disease."

You've now learned a bit about how yoga therapy can help with stress and anxiety. We'll get more deeply into yoga's influence in Part II with the five yogic paths, but first the next chapters demonstrate the influence of beliefs and layers of ourselves (body, life energy/breath, mind/feelings, intellect, and spirit/higher self) on our well-being.

Chapter 2

How Beliefs Result in Stress and Anxiety

Now that you know a bit more about how yoga therapy can help you with stress and anxiety, we will look at one of the fundamental aspects of yoga: how the mind works. In this chapter you will uncover some of your underlying beliefs that cause stress and anxiety. We will examine their historical roots by relating them to past experiences, programming, and brain science. Yogic concepts combine with modern psychology and neuroscience. Practical exercises guide you into shifting your beliefs away from stress and anxiety. It is a process of relating neutral, external experiences to who you really are beyond the old programming and mental habits. This chapter empowers you to literally "change your mind" about stress and anxiety!

What Do You Believe?

Read the following words, pausing after each one and noticing your reaction to it. Gardening. Cooking. Running. Redecorating. Training the dog. People who enjoy these hobbies go to them whenever they can, love doing them, and lose track of time while engaging in the process. People who do not enjoy these hobbies react negatively at the very thought of them. For example, gardeners smile at the dirt under their fingernails because it reminds them of being close to nature. Conversely, folks who would love to let others do all their garden chores think that dirt under the fingernails is unhygienic and could get into the body through the mouth or a cut, which could lead to disease. These people believe that dirt is dirty. A gardener, on the other hand, would tell you that dirt is gold because if there is dirt to grow food, we will never starve. So what you start to see is that in the same situation, depending on our beliefs about dirt under the fingernails, people will have different reactions in response to what we think dirt under the fingernails causes. The same is so for most of our beliefs in life. Many of us are not fully aware of the beliefs that guide our fundamental interactions with life.

What Are Beliefs?

When we consider beliefs in relation to stress, they tend to be ideas about the truth of situations. The gardener believes that dirt contains microbes that support human life. The non-gardener believes that dirt contains germs that may be dangerous to life. Based on a personal belief, one's behavior will be radically different from another's. Hindus believe that the Ganges River is holy and they drink the polluted waters. Few become ill from a river that most scientists believe is fiercely contaminated with a multitude of harmful germs. Beliefs are very strong conveyers of action and reaction and since life is constantly changing, our beliefs usually lag behind.

The wise person knows that beliefs are based on past experience and not always relevant to the present. Such a person is free from anxiety and holds beliefs like the ones below. Notice how the corresponding feeling associated with these beliefs is peacefulness or acceptance.

- All things are changing.
- All emotions pass, including stress and anxiety.
- Change in life brings the need to adapt or work even when we are retired.
- Curiosity embraces the unknown future with joy.
- Patience decreases many modern stresses.

- Constant practice and self-care support a joyful life.
- Listening is important because the human mind is limited.
- Compassion in the face of negativity is helpful because the angry person is hurting.

We have been raised in a fast-paced world where our beliefs may compound that stress. Modern beliefs approach life in an externally focused manner. Notice how each of the following beliefs about life is out of the believer's control. These views of life lead to stress and later to anxiety.

- I love to have all of my favorite things around me.
- A big, beautiful home equals a happy life.
- I eat this because it tastes good.
- Success is reflected in promotions and pay raises.
- Attractive people are better people.
- Doing everything for my family means they will like me.
- Going to a fancy restaurant in new clothing garners respect.
- I love to give my kids everything they need to be happy, so we join every activity and go on as many vacations as possible.
- I need this new item so I will just charge it.

Yoga teaches that all situations in life are neutral. It is the mind that creates value judgments based on likes and dislikes, personal desires, expectations, family values, and cultural assumptions. It is common to feel burdened and have emotional reactions to problems when, in fact, a problem is merely a problem. In order to alleviate anxiety around problems, we must uncover our beliefs. Any limiting belief will cause some kind of stress and ultimately anxiety. We shift stress from a burden to a path of self-realization by discovering the belief patterns that bring acceptance to all situations, whether they are problematic or not.

Where Do Beliefs Come From?

We create beliefs from many places from early on in life. Once we have core beliefs established, usually by the age of eight or ten years old, we filter our information and events into our preexisting beliefs. Without being conscious of the process, we actually seek to prove those beliefs correct and give more psychological weight to experiences that confirm what we already believe. Unless we excavate these beliefs, as we will do throughout this book, we continue to compile evidence and instill our beliefs more deeply—whether they serve our well-being or not!

Early on, we learned what to believe from those we spent the most time with, such as teachers and family. These beliefs include what we were overtly taught in terms of values, but also what we were covertly taught through observing and mirroring behaviors. On a broader scale, society socialized us through media and interactions with friends and acquaintances. From a personal perspective, meaningful experiences also shaped our beliefs. These impact experiences may have come in the form of achievements or losses. The following exercise examines an early anxiety impact experience to help you begin to uproot the associated beliefs.

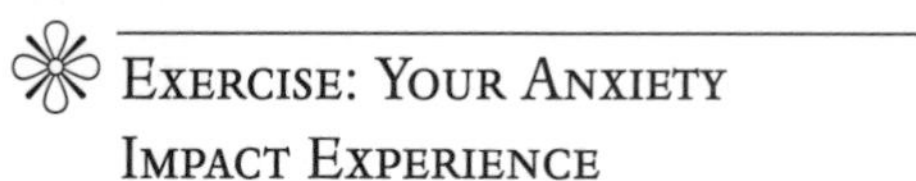

Exercise: Your Anxiety Impact Experience

1. Recall the first time you remember being stressed or anxious. This need not *actually* be the first time it happened; just trace as far back in your mind as you can right now and select an early experience.
2. Remember as much as possible about this past moment of anxiety. Where were you? What was happening? Who was with you? How did they respond to your worries?
3. Do your best to remember what was occurring inside you as well. This exercise is for you alone; it is okay if you do not remember clearly. Trust what comes up for you, as that is likely beneficial information right now. During this early anxiety experience, what thoughts do you remember thinking?

What bodily sensations did you feel? How were you breathing? What emotions surfaced? What were you worried would happen? It may be beneficial to journal these observations to get them out of your head.

Self-Perception and Early Programming

It is important to instill a sense of personal values and empathy in children if we are to enjoy a healthy society. However, not all socialization winds up being healthy for children. This isn't because those doing the socializing are bad people; often, although they did their best, they did not have the skills to be completely supportive or kind in how they conveyed social norms. Negative or abusive instruction can damage the fragile self-image of children. Often people who have anxiety were taught with some negativity, such as punishment, coldness, or perfectionism. This can lead to us questioning our value as people or feeling enormous pressure over things that in the long run don't matter. This early programming shapes how we perceive and respond to the world around us as well as understand who we are. Just like most computer programs run behind the scenes while we enjoy the front-end effects, so early beliefs govern us, unnoticed, while self-perception and the action of life take place in the conscious realm.

Exercise: Who am I?

Through the processes of early programming affecting our self-image, we discern who we are and who we are not. Many of us get invested in this self-perception, clinging rigidly to some attributes where it may benefit us to be more flexible. Furthermore, yoga philosophy teaches that who we truly are cannot be defined, and connecting to this higher, ineffable self is soothing and enlightening.

1. List some of the ways you define yourself. Include features like family roles, personality attributes, relationships, physical characteristics, community, education, work, political and religious affiliations, possessions, and so on.

2. Review your list and circle the three items you most identify yourself with. What, specifically, are you identifying with?
3. Note which parts of these roles, characteristics, or affiliations change. Which aspects are unchanging?
4. How do you understand *yourself* in each of these roles?

Higher Self Perception

Yoga offers a means of understanding how the mind works and acknowledges that wrong beliefs cause suffering. Yoga views ignorance as the root of emotional pain. Ignorance in this case is not an academic unknowing; rather, it is being ignorant of the higher self in everyday situations. Most of us live as if our small ego selves and the ever-changing material reality are all that exists. Yoga, although not a religion, teaches us to have faith in an unchanging aspect of reality or higher aspect of self that transcends the ego. If we think that we are only a body, we fret over protecting the physical self. If we are mainly concerned with image and being likeable, we worry about what others think. However, if we value the higher self first and foremost, the changing aspects of our lives such as appearance, money, and social status are less likely to create stress. By freeing ourselves from ignorance, we transcend our programmed beliefs and meet both pain and pleasure with a peaceful state of mind. Thus, in yoga therapy, we shift to a spiritual view of reality through balance in the mind, education, and lifestyle changes.

As we grow to understand ourselves, we come to realize that even our belief systems change over time. As we align our beliefs with the higher self, we remove ignorance. The body's systems, such as the autonomic nervous system and the three brains discussed in the previous chapter, respond to this shift and anxiety is lessened. By appreciating our deeper spiritual beliefs on an ongoing basis, we are able to remain neutral, thus removing stress from life and expressing well-being throughout the day.

Exercise: Accessing the Higher Self

The more you understand specific aspects of your higher self, the more readily you will remove ignorance from your everyday thoughts and beliefs. The following exercise offers a path to realizing more about your spiritual self.

1. When are you most like yourself? What activities, states of mind, or personal characteristics help you feel at your best? When is your behavior in alignment with the highest version of yourself? Note that you don't have to be good at these activities or comfortable in the situations. The feeling you are seeking is one of honesty and openness. When are you expressing "This is who I AM"?
2. Express these activities, states of mind, or characteristics. Journal, list, draw, or collage images that remind you of your true, higher self. When you know the situations, thoughts, and traits that resonate most clearly with your higher self, you are able to seek them out. They become skills that help you cope with and eventually transform your stress.

Science of Belief and Anxiety

"It is all in your head!" We are familiar with that phrase. It is insulting if you have stress or anxiety as it says, "I don't believe you actually have any stress!" Imagine you interpreted the phrase as "Due to your anxiety, your brain has actually changed so that you can identify your stress more easily. Your brain is so clever!" This is actually what happens in the brains of people who have had stress or anxiety for a long time. The brain gets more attentive to it.

The brain looks for stress because it tries to protect us from it. Longstanding beliefs create deep neural connections in the brain, which can ultimately prevent anxious people from controlling the anxiety. This process of neuroplasticity, or the changing shape of the brain, has been well studied in chronic pain patients. In people with chronic pain, the brain gets so vigilant that a bigger part of the brain is focused on the painful area of the body. The nerve synapses transmitting the pain impulses to the brain get more efficient. The brain even *decreases* its ability to intercept and modulate the pain. Therefore, the more we look for pain, the more pain we feel and the better we are physically able to experience it! The process is similar with emotional pain, stress, and anxiety, based on your internal focus and beliefs. Chronic stress changes the shape and function of the brain. When we look at it this way, yes, it is "all in your head"—because you have such a wonderful brain that you have managed to change its structure.

Stress can come on without any conscious awareness of what triggered it. Most of us have had the experience of suddenly remembering a person or situation and feeling deeply and instantly good or bad. A song, a voice, or some other environmental trigger activates something in the brain and the neural pathway fires automatically. It is the same for stress and anxiety. When we are in a situation or perceive something through the senses that has previously caused anxiety, the brain, in its wisdom, follows that neural pathway leading to a sense of stress and anxiety. If we then have the belief, based on previous experiences, that we are helpless over the current situation then the only choice is to experience the negative effects of stress and anxiety. Conversely, if we believe that we have a certain amount of control over the situation then we can also control our response to the anxiety we experience. Research is clear that whether the stress occurs at work, in relationships, or in sports, people who have the belief that they possess some power over the situation experience less negative stress and anxiety.

Know that your brain can change! Your brain is there to protect you. You have a phenomenal brain. It is just that sometimes the brain is doing too good a job protecting you from possible future problems, so anxiety sets in. The structures of your brain have changed to make you hypervigilant to situations and external things that might cause stress or anxiety. Since the brain is changeable it can also become less attentive to the adverse conditions around you; however, beliefs about what causes the stress and anxiety also need to change. The next time you feel anxious, realize that it is really your brain that has become overly vigilant.

There is no life-threatening emergency, it's just old programming affecting the internal world because the brain is overly sensitive. When you change your beliefs about and response to stress and anxiety, your brain will once again change its structure. This moves you toward calm responses to what were once perceived as stressful situations.

Exercise: Thought Patterns

We are often not aware of the underlying beliefs that drive our emotions and behaviors. Yoga therapy seeks the roots of harming beliefs. Through self-examination, yoga therapy supports you in weeding out flawed beliefs and adapting harmful emotions and behaviors, thereby creating permanent internal and external change. By monitoring your thoughts in a systematic way, you can learn more about the automatic habits of your mind and become conscious of how to change them.

1. Set a timer to ring at frequent intervals, no less than 10 minutes and no more than 40.
2. When the timer rings, hear the last thought that was in your mind and jot it down. You may add details like time of day or activity. More detail will help you discern patterns and reveal underlying beliefs. Some passing thoughts might be, "Thinking about lunch," "Rehearsing conversation with belligerent coworker. Feeling worried. Supposed to be doing data entry," or "Remembering last night's game. Wishing I was still playing the sport but am too tired. Procrastinating cold calls."
3. With regular practice of this exercise, you will have great insight into your nonconscious thoughts and your overall relationship with yourself. Pay special attention to repetitive messages and points of view within your own mind. Remember: your inner world creates your life experience. How do your everyday thoughts contribute to your anxiety or sense of well-being?

4. Once you understand your patterns you can work to change them. Is there a new thought you could use whenever you become aware of the anxiety habit in your thinking? Continue working through this and the next chapter for other specific exercises to transform stressful and anxious beliefs.

Attitude (*Bhava*) Alters the Situation

The Yoga Institute in Mumbai offers many classic teaching stories to help students understand how to apply yoga philosophy. The following story shows how our beliefs and thoughts color our days and can build us into the person we are in the world.

Once upon a time a drought thrust an ancient kingdom into chaos. With the ground crusty and brittle, farmers could not tend the fields. Trouble ensued as some farmers took to gambling and others to theft. Fortunately the king was wise and had enough grain stored to feed his people and an idea for a project to busy their idle hands. The king declared that all unemployed farmers were to begin building a temple.

Farmers started their work at a quarry in the hot sun, swinging heavy mallets and crushing stone to build the foundation of the temple. The king's anthropologist documented this endeavor by interviewing the farmers-turned-stonecutters. He asked the first farmer what he was doing.

The first farmer said, "Can't you see? I am stuck in this hot sun because of this awful drought. I am forced to crack stone like a prisoner; ours is a cursed kingdom."

The anthropologist approached a clean-cut man who worked methodically and asked the same question, "What are you doing?"

The second farmer replied, "To earn my food ration I am working eight hours a day cutting stone, sir. I can support my family this way. Do I receive a bonus for sharing my views with you?"

Lastly, the anthropologist went to another and asked again, "What are you doing?" This man continued cutting his stone until he reached a natural stopping point.

He placed the mallet down, walked to the anthropologist and said, "Can't you see, friend? I am building a temple." The anthropologist concluded that outwardly, all three farmers were cracking stone, yet their states of mind varied greatly.

In this story, the third man was the only individual who was working with his higher self in mind. He was in the same situation as the others but felt completely different about it. Because of his self-reliance, he did not allow external forces such as others' requirements of him or money to control how he felt about what he was doing. He believed in his duty to perform responsibilities in a manner that maintains mental peace. Our attitude toward a situation alters the situation itself.

You can see from the story of the temple-building farmers how beliefs create the reality of a situation. The first temple builder believed he was enslaved—by the drought, by the work, by the directive of the king, and worst of all by his own sense of meaninglessness—which is the opposite of yoga, connecting to the freedom of the higher self. The second temple builder also showed a sense of powerlessness but had some hope of working his way out of the impoverished situation. The third temple builder was present without a wish for things to be different. He showed a belief in the meaning of his efforts and did his best at the job in front of him, even though it was not his chosen career. He was connected to his higher self and believed that he was a part of something greater; thus, he was at peace with the situation. The moral of the story is that our viewpoint determines the process and personal outcome of a situation. The same external activity may have completely different internal outcomes based solely on our beliefs.

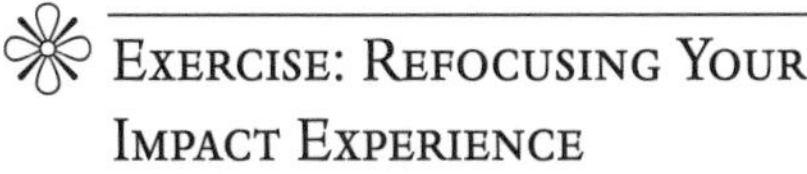

Exercise: Refocusing Your Impact Experience

Use this exercise to help you shift your beliefs about a situation. The impactful experiences of our childhoods instill beliefs so deeply within us that we may not be conscious of when we are seeing a current situation through an old lens. Just like the temple builders, you can transform a current stressful situation into something neutral by decoding the old programming and connecting more deeply inward, to the higher self.

1. List ten activities that you find connecting or uplifting. How are these events positive? What beliefs, thoughts, and emotions do you bring to them? What spiritual feelings, or virtues, are strengthened? For example, cooks find inspiration and peace of mind through that work. They enjoy the kitchen sounds and the smells and textures of food. While it is useful to provide meals for yourself and loved ones, the real enjoyment lies in the creativity. To take this understanding to the next level, realize that any creative activity may be soothing to the cook's soul, whether it takes place in the kitchen or not. Cooking is simply one of many activities that connects to the virtue of creativity.
2. List a few stressful events of the last week. Choose one impactful stress experience from this list to work with. How was this situation different than the positive events you listed in Step 1? Which thoughts and emotions arose? What beliefs were present? Notice that the stress was not only from what was happening around you but also from the internal story.
3. Rewrite the programming of your own story through playing with your beliefs. What spiritual feelings or virtues could you cultivate while engaging in this stressful situation? How could these virtues transform the event into an opportunity for personal growth? Allow the perspective of the third temple-builder to uplift you as you find meaning in all tasks, remembering that the situation itself is neutral.

Exercise: Meeting the Inner Anthropologist

Anthropologists, like the one in the temple builders story, study human origins, thought, and behavior. They are researchers who approach their subjects with genuine interest, appreciation, and reverence, free from judgment. These objective observers possess a deep desire to understand the underlying beliefs of cultures that contributed to their development. Similarly, throughout this book, we ask you to take the compassionate, curious stance of an anthropologist as you study the origins of your stress.

1. Considering yourself as an anthropologist—curious, nonjudgmental, and objective—what have you observed about your inner culture of beliefs?
2. Which beliefs and perspectives are most prevalent in your internal culture? When facing them objectively, do you agree with them all?
3. Note the beliefs that create a culture of stress and anxiety within you.
4. Which beliefs are important to you now? Which ones align with your current values system and spiritual intention?
5. What new insights arise from your objective look at your beliefs? Which ones are you ready to discard? What beliefs and perspectives do you wish to strengthen within yourself? How can these help you cope with stress, anxiety, and associated destructive thoughts, emotions, and beliefs?
6. Choose one helpful belief and apply it to stressful situations over the next week.

Modern Psychotherapy, Anxiety, and Yoga

The science of modern psychology directly relates to many fundamental yoga concepts. Yoga's ancient philosophies and techniques are sometimes repackaged for a modern world, but their roots and outcomes are the same. Yoga therapy incorporates, and transcends, the techniques applied in popular modern psychotherapeutic models. Notice the similarities between the psychological counseling techniques listed below and traditional yoga.

Cognitive-Behavioral Therapy

Cognitive-Behavioral Therapy (CBT) is a popular counseling method that addresses the thoughts and cognitive processes behind unwanted behaviors or emotions. By changing the thoughts, we can change the feelings and reactions to them. Mindfulness-Based Cognitive Therapy (MBCT) adds training in witnessing the passing thoughts and feelings with acceptance, so clients learn to separate themselves from their thoughts. This process of witnessing the contents of the mind and shifting them to a more truthful, uplifted frame is a strong aspect of classical yoga and Comprehensive Yoga Therapy. Like CBT and MBCT, yoga therapy teaches you to witness, accept, and confront unhealthy thoughts and beliefs, replacing them with more objective thoughts. Many of the exercises in this book teach you to do this.

Rational-Emotive Therapy

Rational-Emotive Therapy (RET) is a precursor to CBT whereby clients are asked to evaluate the rationality of their thoughts and perceptions. Similar to the yogic practices we do in this book, like sense mastery and concentration, RET directs clients toward self-enquiry. Through RET they address their unrealistic expectations and flawed beliefs, allowing a realistic world view which, in turn, limits painful emotional reactions. Yoga therapy works as RET and will teach you to view yourself and situations more objectively, through a realistic, rather than personally biased, frame.

Solution-Focused Brief Therapy

Solution-Focused Brief Therapy (SFBT) is the counseling model adopted by most employee health plans. As in yoga therapy, clients and therapists work together in SFBT to clearly define outcome goals and action steps to move in that direction. Similarly, many exercises throughout this book ask you to look at what small steps you can take in the direction of becoming more like your vision of your higher self. Simple, everyday changes have a rapid and powerful effect on our quality of life. SFBT is a form of positive psychology, which does not talk about people's problems; rather, as its name suggests, it focuses on moving forward with solutions. As with SFBT, yoga therapy is collaborative and supports you in taking action toward specific positive goals.

Exercise: Belief Determines Outcomes

1. Earlier in this chapter, you worked with the first anxiety experience you could remember. If you could go back in time, as your adult self, to the moment of that impact experience, what would you tell your young self? How would you offer comfort and reassurance?
2. Knowing what your younger self was thinking and feeling at the time, what new perspective could you offer? Is there an alternative to your belief system of that past time?
3. Record these comforting sentiments, as they may soothe your grown-up anxiety, too! Shape them into affirmations and apply them as autosuggestions to transform your underlying core beliefs. Notice how this process is similar to modern psychological approaches.

You Can Create Your Current Beliefs

At any point in our lives and yoga journeys, we may encounter obstacles (*klesas*) that prohibit us from thoroughly experiencing the mind, no matter what level of clarity we have. Sometimes we believe our own thoughts and think they are an accurate representation of reality. We have this idea that if we think something, then that is the way it is. Not true. Usually, what we think has very little to do with the present situation and almost everything to do with filtering the present through past beliefs.

Here is a breakdown of the process: An impact experience happened. The mind kicked in and interpreted the emotional input using the language of thoughts. These interpretations solidified into beliefs which continually filtered new experiences through the old impact experience. We get stuck with stress because we persist in interpreting things through this old filter.

As we grow more intimate with our mental states and thought patterns, we understand that these filters, or beliefs, are impermanent and subject to change. We do not identify with our thoughts and emotions, and we recognize that they are just passing through. We begin to experience the linguistic component of thoughts and how language creates and conditions how we will ultimately experience things. There is a difference between "I'm angry!" and "I'm experiencing anger right now." In the first example, we identify ourselves *as* anger; in the second, there is some distance between the emotion and who we are. Note how often (and unmindfully) we say, "I have to ..." instead of "I'm going to ..." or "I choose to ..." Do you see how the first choice of words limits your perception of freedom and self-direction? What would happen if you thought of going to work in a snowstorm as an adventure, rather than a great inconvenience or threatening situation? Language choices impact our beliefs. As our beliefs change, the external situation seems to as well.

Often the clear mind has been described as a pure bright sky, unobstructed by clouds. Our thoughts, and the reactive behavior patterns that result from them, cover up this radiant awareness. Sometimes the cloud cover is thin or sparse, but at other times the sky is blackened by raging storm clouds: thoughts that are confusing or have enormous emotional impact. The Thought Patterns exercise (see page 45) helps you see the clouds for what they are: mental constructs. You become clear on how certain beliefs limit you, how they constrict your perceptions, and how you can choose to let go of those beliefs and live with greater freedom. Gradually, with the ability to see things clearly, the clouds of old belief start thinning and eventually evaporate. This then heralds the beginning of true wisdom. By witnessing your passing thoughts without attaching to them, you begin to navigate life with greater freedom, ease, and confidence in your ability to choose wisely and from higher perspective, released from the strain of old programming.

Exercise: Thought Awareness

In order to keep the mind still and focused on the present moment, we must release our emotional attachment to our wandering thoughts and day-to-day tribulations. Many of us are well-trained at removing ourselves from our bodies, internal sensations, and mental activities as a means to block them out. In yoga, detached awareness is more like taking a step back from experiences rather than blocking them out. Apply this exercise to help gain some objective distance from your thoughts so that you can understand them—and yourself—a little better.

1. The next time you feel stressed, instead of splitting yourself off from what is happening inside or making it or yourself "go away," simply become a more neutral witness inside of yourself.
2. Continue to feel physical sensations and emotions. Watch your mind as it continues to interpret and chatter, but witness this process without involvement, as if you were watching a movie.
3. Acknowledge each thought and feeling as it occurs, and allow it to pass, thus witnessing a more complete view of what is happening inside. Imagine these thoughts and feelings passing through your consciousness the way clouds pass through the sky on a warm, breezy day. From this awareness, we learn to know and trust ourselves and respond from a place of self-understanding and connection.

Exercise: Tension Awareness

Similar to the exercise on Thought Awareness, you may observe how stress and anxiety impact your physical self. The state of mind is revealed through the body. Our thoughts and attitudes are reflected in our postures, both in yoga poses and how we carry ourselves through the world. Likewise, physical posture and health reflect on the state of the mind. Anxiety often manifests in the body with quick, erratic movements, trembling hands, and a tight, high-pitched voice, which further draw the mind and senses out of balance. Conversely, when we relax the body, the mind follows suit. We become less mentally agitated and feel better equipped to face the challenges of our day. Once you are aware of your habits of holding tension, you can consciously suggest these areas relax throughout the day and even tailor your yoga posture practice to support that physical relaxation.

1. The next time you are stressed or anxious, notice how your body holds the tension. Pay close attention to the tightening of specific muscles, aches, or a sense of being limited.
2. Health care practitioners sometimes use a diagram of a human figure to mark the areas and qualities of pain and injury. Modify this idea by drawing an outline of your own figure. Color the body to indicate areas of stress. Be creative, using color or texture to represent different sensations. The top three common areas to hold stress are neck, lower back, and jaw. Forehead, eyes, stomach, bottom, toes, and fists are also well-known for housing stress. Any area of your body can hold your anxiety; remain open and curious.

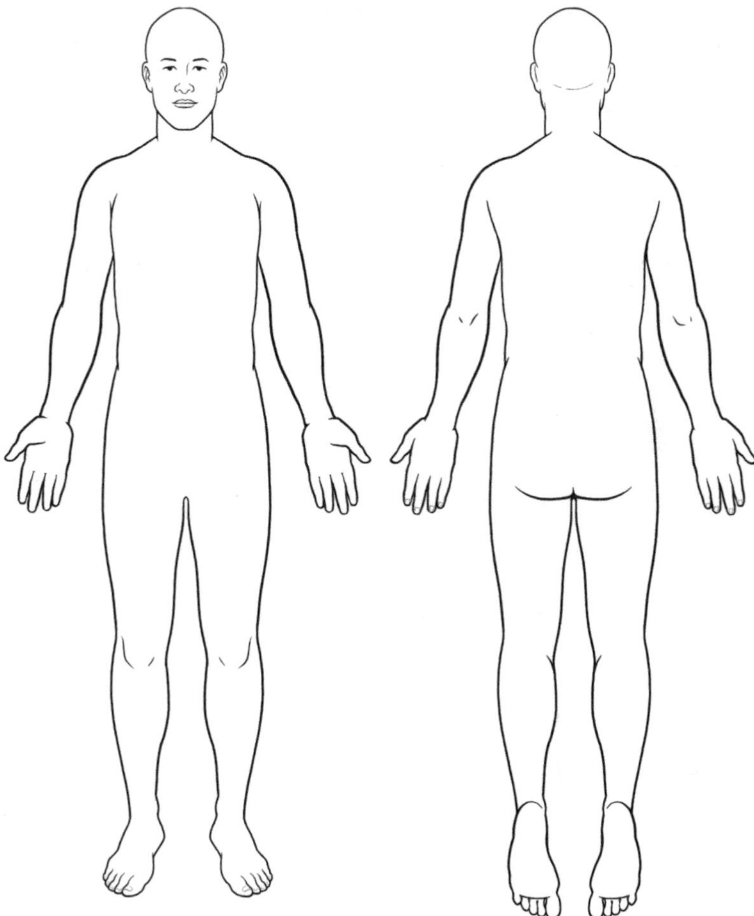

Figure 2.1: Diagram of a human figure to mark areas and qualities of pain and injury

3. Breathe deeply, with a small smile on your face, and suggest to these tense areas, "Relax … reeelaaaax …" You may repeat the creative exercise to depict the difference relaxation has made in your body.

Thank you for exploring your past and enquiring into your current beliefs and patterns. Knowing where your habits come from is a key step in claiming your power to shift your life in uplifting directions. Through examining your history, cultivating internal awareness, and making distinct and conscious choices, you are moving yourself away from stress and anxiety already!

Chapter Summary

1. It is possible to remove stress from a person, although life circumstances may require effort.
2. All situations in life are neutral. It is the mind that judges and interprets them.
3. Recognize your beliefs about life and who you are. Gradually alter them through awareness to be more uplifting and true.
4. Beliefs guide our fundamental interactions with life.
5. Early programming governs how we perceive, understand, and respond to ourselves and the world around us, whether we are conscious of these underlying beliefs or not.
6. The beliefs that cause suffering are on a different level of perception than the thoughts that offer internal freedom. Who we truly are or what life is really about cannot be defined. Connecting to this higher, ineffable self and perspective of life is soothing and enlightening.
7. Yoga views ignorance of the higher self or ever-present divine as the root of emotional pain.
8. Repetitive stressful beliefs and anxious feelings change the shape and function of the brain to make you more sensitive to stress. Observing and shifting thoughts, beliefs, and physical reactions to external circumstances can reshape the brain to function in a more relaxed state.
9. By taking ownership of the beliefs that create stress and replacing them with a spiritual perspective, all aspects of life become more fulfilling.
10. Yoga therapy incorporates ancient philosophies and techniques, which are echoed in popular modern psychotherapeutic models.

11. Through the process of awareness, you have the power to move your thoughts and physical reactions in the direction of relaxation and ease.

Throughout this chapter, you have gained awareness of your underlying beliefs and the effect they have in your everyday life. Continue with the practices that counterprogram your stress and anxiety. You are shifting your beliefs so that they reflect who you really are! In the next chapter we build on your awareness and delve into the places where you may not be as aware, thereby shining light into the darker corners so they may be properly cleaned out.

Chapter 3
Redefine Your Beliefs

This chapter explores your underlying beliefs and helps free you from the tyranny of fearful assumptions and worried projections. Go deeper into your inner world in order to realize how your beliefs shape your life without you even knowing! We offer perspectives that shift beliefs and help you perceive the world in a more peaceful, neutral way. As you gain insight into the driving beliefs below the surface of consciousness, the exercises of this chapter support you in neutralizing them. This redefinition of your beliefs changes your experience of reality so that stress and anxiety loosen their grip and a feeling of ease is the new normal. The first step is to become conscious of what upsets your inner peace. Then notice how you react to those things. By understanding what is really important to you and the effects of those things on your state of mind, you will begin to redefine your own reactions to what happens *outside* of you by managing your *internal* world.

Digging into the Not-Conscious

Lee was a marketing executive who knew a lot about the way people's minds work and what they want. Before attending yoga classes, Lee rarely turned that knowledge inward, instead applying it to manipulating others and "winning the game of life." When Lee was laid off after twenty years with the company, the realization landed that Lee's relationship was in shambles, the children were independent teenagers, and the extended family a mere afterthought. Worst of all, Lee had no idea how to cope with the sense of loss and self-image issues that followed the layoff. It was time for a change and, on the advice of a friend, Lee began taking yoga classes and quickly realized that this life's priorities had never been healthy. With work always coming first, family and even self-care were rarely attended. Lee was simply not conscious of the priorities expressing themselves through everyday choices. Through conscious self-inquiry and small, daily adjustments, Lee learned to express deeper beliefs and priorities and put self-care first, which opened the door to greater connection and enjoyment with the family.

The conscious mind can't know everything; hence, faith in a larger reality is necessary. Without this faith, the personality pursues futile attempts to control reality; trying to do the impossible is very stressful. It is important, as you uncover uncomfortable ideas or flaws in your personality, to keep an open mind and remain diligent. Be aware that your ideas and what you perceive as flaws are there because at some point in time they were helpful to you. Some of these habits may not be helpful to you anymore; they might actually be getting in the way of you living your life to the fullest. Be kind to yourself and just observe, knowing that you developed them because they served you in certain situations. You are on a path of discovery about the patterns, thoughts, and behaviors that influence your anxiety. One of the intentions of this book is to free you from stress by connecting with a sense of something more in all areas of life. True connection requires a shift in thinking and a willingness to investigate attitudes and beliefs. Honest evaluation of your present attitude toward stress is essential. Once we acknowledge frustrations, weaknesses, and fears, we are open to new patterns of behavior. Breakthroughs, new ideas, and profound insights are norms as we bring yoga practice into everyday life through expanding awareness.

Most of us live within a narrow band of awareness. We go through similar routines every day, associating with others who hold similar beliefs and expectations. What passes through conscious awareness is a mere fraction of what is going on within us. An iceberg reveals only its tip above the water, while its mass hides below the surface. Our consciousness is like the iceberg. Memories, knowledge, hopes, expectations, thought patterns, feelings, sensory impressions, and the like reside almost entirely beneath the surface of our awareness. In psychological language there is *unconscious*, lacking the capacity for perception as in deep sleep, and *nonconscious*, that which is beyond awareness; specific psychologists have bred even more connotations into these two words. To avoid confusion, we combine these ideas in the word "not-conscious" so that we may incorporate dreams, unacknowledged beliefs, and other mental processes that exist below the surface of awareness. As we understand more about our consciousness, both what we are aware of and what is not-conscious, we become effective at shifting our beliefs about reality. Since it is difficult to access not-conscious material, the task of knowing ourselves stretches across a lifetime.

Exercise: Considering Priorities

The following brainstorming exercise will give you insight into what you *think* is important versus what you *believe* is important. In order to avoid biasing you, we do not give any examples of what a person's priorities might be. To get the most out of this brainstorming exercise, allow yourself the freedom of free association—in other words, just write what comes to mind. Your honest, unfiltered, and undirected responses will offer the greatest insight and reveal important action steps as you consider what is most important to you right now.

1. List your top ten priorities in life. Don't think too much about it; just ask yourself "What is most important to me?" and start writing. Be honest and do not filter as you simply jot these things down off the top of your head. Do any of your answers surprise you?
2. Since this was a brainstorming exercise, you may have thought of your priorities out of order. Reread your list and rank the items from most to least important. How many items did you

list before you recorded what is *actually* the highest priority in your life?

3. Is your physical, energetic, emotional, intellectual, or spiritual health on the list anywhere? When we put our own health first, we are in a strong position to transform stress. Who, what, or which tasks are top on your list?
4. Set this list aside. We will review it in the exercise Playing with Perception and Reality, later in this chapter.

Awareness

Comprehensive Yoga Therapy teaches that suffering is a state of mind; thus, healing begins in the mind. Reality itself is neutral. Typically, the beliefs that underlie our stress and anxiety exist in the not-conscious realm but are expressed through everyday situations. Most people lack the awareness to challenge these automatic lines of thinking, let alone delve into their not-conscious roots. For a moment, let us notice how there are options in our state of mind toward reality. Consider the chart below:

Stressful Reaction to Reality	*Neutral Observation of Reality*
That person is so rude.	Rude behavior externalizes one's own suffering.
Traffic is brutal.	Traffic slows down driving times.
Deadlines are so much pressure.	Deadlines reveal organization.
There is too much on my list.	I act upon the most important thing. When complete, I move on to the next.
Reality controls me so I am out of control.	Reality is neutral so I feel at peace with things.

How we react to reality is a choice. This major tenet of classical yoga teaches that all situations in life are, in fact, unbiased. It is the mind that creates value judgments based on personal desires, expectations, and cultural assumptions. Generally, we understand that when people are emotionally reactive to a problem they feel burdened. Ironically, healthy reactions such as neutrality and acceptance are often met with confusion. The truth is, a problem is merely a problem, a pain in life is simply pain—no reactions required. The psychological component of yoga therapy helps unearth the not-conscious so that we understand our reactions more deeply. Any underlying limiting beliefs or unresolved emotions will cause stress and anxiety. When we begin to understand what is not-conscious, we neutralize what was unresolved. We minimize stress by not reacting to a problem. Once we are in the pattern of accepting reality, our "problems" shift from burdens to a path to the higher self.

By practicing calm awareness, we cultivate an objective and nonjudgmental attitude to everyday life. Freed from the internal tyranny of preconceived perceptions and beliefs, we are able to accept each moment as it comes, without the stress of it not meeting expectations or the anxiety of how it may turn out in the future. In the beginning, bring awareness at least once daily to one of the stressful items on the list from the following exercise, Conscious Self-Inquiry. Notice your breathing as you sit in traffic or when someone cuts in front of you at the store. Observe your emotions during and after a difficult conversation with a loved one or coworker. Pause for just a moment before responding to someone else's criticism. These are all very simple yet profound awareness actions that can dramatically start to alter your stress. Thoughts don't just "happen"; we can choose them. Acknowledge underlying patterns of belief and create new thought patterns. Ultimately, awareness alters how your mind processes daily events.

Exercise: Conscious Self-Inquiry

What we're trying to do with the exercises in this book is help you reduce your stress by taking things that are out of control and interpreting them in a way that will help you. Awareness gives you control over your inner world. It's normal to worry about things we don't control. There could be an earthquake tomorrow, a child could crash the bike, someone could lose a job … and if we spend a lot of time worrying about tomorrow, we turn stress to anxiety. However, if we go through the day with awareness, we can hold on to peace of mind. We will feel faith and comfort even if we don't know what's coming. Try this exercise to help you with that.

1. Throughout the day, pick random moments and record your current thoughts and feelings. The more randomized this is, the more you will understand your patterns as you observe what is present in different situations. Acknowledging thoughts and feelings without judging them is an important step in building awareness. You began to practice something similar to this in the previous chapter.
2. You can broaden this internal awareness of what is truly happening beneath the surface through a process of gentle self-inquiry. Become curious about your inner world. Simply let yourself breathe and observe how your mind follows and reacts to your breath. Do not control the breath or what the mind is doing, simply witness what occurs in your thoughts and feelings as you breathe naturally.
3. This seemingly simple practice is in fact essential for preparing your mind for deeper awareness down the road. The mind's tendency is to relate itself to things in the outer world. A scattered mind preoccupied with the external realm will never be able to focus and start looking inward. Reassociation of the mind's focus is initiated by a smooth, steady, and equal breath. This type of yogic breathing causes minimal mental distraction. When the breath is erratic, choppy, or gasping, it comes as no surprise that the mind is easily disrupted—the agitated sound and physical motion draw the mind away from the inner state.
4. As an ongoing practice, become aware of your inner world through recording thoughts and feelings; remain aware of it through a smooth breath.

Perceptions

To begin to foster this awareness of how your mind behaves, evaluate how much peace you experience in your daily life and routine. Hopefully there are moments of sanctuary: eating meals with the family, taking brief walks, during exercise. But what happens when you leave these environments? How does your mind react to waking up a bit late or to sitting in heavy traffic? Reflect on your relationships with an irascible boss or that coworker or client who gets on your last nerve. How do you handle situations when things do not quite go as you planned, at work or with other daily chores and activities? What about your relationships with those close to you: your family members, spouse or partner, children, dear friends?

As you consider these elements of your life, please be honest but avoid ideas of "good" and "bad"—the intent is awareness, not condemnation. If even one or two responses to the above examples were not even-keeled, they likely are rooted in not-conscious beliefs that often manifest as stress. The first step is to become conscious of what upsets your inner peace. Then notice how you react to those things. Remember, stress is nothing more than the environment interacting with us. That interaction is constant. We cannot eliminate the external stressors, but how they affect us is entirely under our control. We diminish stress by being self-reliant in reworking beliefs and learning to respond, rather than react, to the external world.

What You Perceive, You Believe (Whether It's Real or Not!)

While spending some time on a beach vacation, one of our Comprehensive Yoga Therapists was disturbed by a yappy dog across the street. Even a little thing like a dog can turn a vacation into a different kind of situation. Even after years of yoga practice, this yogi had to admit that the sound of the dog was annoying. The neighbors put the dog outside while relaxing behind closed windows with the air conditioner running while the yogi, with the clean ocean breeze blowing through open windows, received the full effects of the dog's barking. He thought that the yappy dog must also bother the neighbors when they returned from the beach, so they put him outside for peace and quiet. Of course, all the people in the tightly situated row homes were subject to the dog. *Yap! Yap! Yap-yap-yap!*

When the yogi mentioned this idea to a dog-loving relative, she didn't know what he meant. The yogi complained that the ignorant neighbors put their dog outside with no regard for the neighborhood, and his loved one replied, "But that little dog is so cute—look at the way he runs around on their deck. He is just lonely."

Lesson learned. While the yogi thought of barking dogs as an intrusion on personal space, the dog-loving relative found the dog's barking cute. She loves dogs; she loves caring for her dogs at home; she pets unfamiliar dogs in the street. The yogi quickly decided to agree with her and become a fellow dog-lover, thereby releasing any stress. The yapping is just a cute little dog singing his praise to the world. With this new perspective, the yogi bade goodbye to the ignorant neighbor that he created in his mind and said hello to freedom. A deeper example of the same process is described below. This is a common occurrence of how the awareness of deeper beliefs creates a shift within a person's entire approach to life.

Drew, a twenty-six-year-old yoga student, began attending classes with friends. Work was becoming stressful and at the same time, Drew thought more and more about the future, settling down, and taking life seriously. Drew's social circle spent most of their free time going out, drinking, eating on the run, and chatting about pop culture, which was beginning to feel frustrating as Drew contemplated deeper questions about life. Older people in yoga class revealed that they did not think about health until their thirties and spent a lot of years wishing they had taken better care when they were younger. Drew took that lesson to heart and sought a stronger path to health and well-being.

The beginning of Drew's yoga experience was driven by social pressure: following the pack to bars, restaurants, and yoga classes. Soon the personal experience of yoga began to unwind Drew's stress, which elevated perceptions and opened new ways of thinking and alternatives to stressful responses.

Drew's higher self motivated spiritual growth and clarity in order to stay healthy through aging, while everyday perceptions created a lot of stress. Spiritual books and a round of yoga therapy appointments helped Drew connect to a higher self by bringing the yoga off the mat and into work and friendships. Time in yoga classes supported a home practice as well, which grew as Drew realized the days that begin with yoga run much more smoothly. This spurred an interest in a yoga teacher training program. Drew continues to create mental clarity by limiting alcohol and sweets, and appreciates the health and calm these small changes make in daily life. Now Drew's higher self radiates out.

Coping with Change

Two main precepts of yoga psychology help us cope with the fear and anxiety that naturally accompany change. One point relates to the discussion above about the quality of awareness we bring to dealing with the unknown. When we don't know what will happen, it can feel scary or it can feel promising, but the simple reality is that we just don't know! We remove the anxiety when we remain aware that the unknown is simply unknown.

The second point that yoga psychology addresses is that *all things* are changing. Whenever something changes, it automatically disrupts what was happening before that. Even the joy of a great new job is technically a stressful event. The new employee has new responsibilities and even if there is a financial boost, this new way of life can be very different. Change is continual and requires adjustments. Our ability to understand and embrace change will greatly reduce the effect of stress.

The higher self is eternal and constant. By accepting that we do not know everything and that all things are changing, we free ourselves from the common bondage of ignorance, wishing things were different or anticipating a future we cannot know. Unlike matter, which constantly changes, the higher self is constant. Connecting to the higher self, rather than the ever-changing material reality, holds us in a state of calm. Wise people accept that they can't know everything and that all things are changing, then remain peaceful in that awareness. Let's do an exercise that reveals how we examine the unknown and the mysterious future changes that are occurring every day.

Exercise: Playing with Perception and Reality

The story we tell ourselves about a situation has an impact on our stress response to it. Throughout this book, we examine the ways your inner world, belief systems, and habits actually train you to be anxious. This exercise helps unwind the stress habits. From a yoga therapy perspective, the true healing of anxiety happens in the mind and intellect as you connect with awareness of your higher self.

1. List your top ten priorities, such as self-care, children, meditation, career, or hobbies, or reread your final list from the exercise Considering Priorities. Rank your priorities from highest-stress to lowest-stress. What level of stress were the first three items you wrote down? How about the last three items? What does that tell you about your state of mind?
2. After cultivating compassionate awareness of some of the "little things" on your list that stress you out, choose two or three of the most stressful items for further introspection. To get started, here are some examples of "big stressors" that we tend to see:
    - Overworked, too busy, rushed
    - Technology overload
    - Relationship difficulties (boss/coworkers or domestic/family)
    - Constant worry
    - Excessive behaviors (overeating, alcohol consumption, addictions)
    - Insomnia or oversleeping

   You may find it helpful to jot each item atop a piece of paper to give plenty of room to freely explore each point. Fully and honestly work through each of the following questions. For each big stress, note the associated thoughts, feelings, and beliefs. Be honest—it is *your* list and will hopefully start to open you to patterns or behaviors you may not have been aware of at first.

3. What are some beliefs and habits that get in the way of you being able to handle stress (which then might lead to anxiety)? Reflect back on where these beliefs came from and see how they helped you at one point, and might still help you in certain situations. Can you see how in other situations these same beliefs and habits might get in the way?
4. Think of a way to make each of these stressful activities strengthen your state of mind. In other words, how can these stressors remind you of and help you connect to your higher self? Caring for children could strengthen your higher self by allowing you to remember the freedom of playing for its own sake. Thus, caring for kids benefits the adult as much as the child. Work to develop a spiritual virtue, such as patience, discipline, or kindness, via these stressors. Remember, your higher self is the first priority when personal growth is the center of your actions.

We usually see two types of items appear on these lists. The more prevalent type are minor stresses; small irritations that can quickly accumulate throughout the course of a day or week. As these smaller stresses accumulate, the brain does not have time to recover in between the stressors and eventually even a small stressor can cause a large reaction in the person! The awareness exercise above will hopefully assist you in sorting out these nuances from the other type of stresses on your list. It is our sincere hope that this second type, the greater impacting stresses, are fewer in number. We all differ, but depending on our current life situations, some of these stresses may be quite encumbering and detrimental. Being aware of these stresses helps us begin to cope with them, yet a deeper reflection on their root cause helps us understand them on a foundational level.

The roots of our stress may be below the surface of consciousness, yet affect us daily through a nagging sense of mental pressure and physical tension. Old beliefs grow into internal obstacles and subjective states of interpreting and interacting with the world. This personal psychology increases our anxiety, often without our awareness. Yoga's understanding of psychology incorporates the conscious and not-conscious aspects of our internal realms. This consciousness actually includes all physical reality—the body, breath, senses, emotions, ego, and thought processes. Yoga's concept of the mind-body complex demonstrates how ancient psychology considers the mind, body, and spirit as a whole.

There is a lot going on within, and we are barely aware of most of it. Modern use of the word "mind" relates to the intellect and brain. However, yoga defines the concept of mind as mind-body complex (*citta*). Viewing a person holistically means that the body is a part of the mind. Just as the nervous system reaches from the brain to every muscle, organ, and gland in the body, so our thoughts, feelings, sensory input, and connection to spirit affect us physically. Note this includes beliefs and emotions that lie below the surface of our awareness. By noticing the state of the physical body, you may gain clues about your emotions and beliefs. When there is tension in the body, the mind will be stressed; an anxious mind is reflected in the body. Mind and matter relate to each other.

Both matter and the mind are continuously changing, which is an unstable state of existence. The higher self is eternal and constant. In yoga philosophy, matter is defined as all things perceived by consciousness. One main feature of matter is that it is constantly changing. The constituents of nature (*gunas*), which will be discussed further in Chapter 7, are active (*rajasic*), inactive (*tamasic*), and balanced (*sattvic*). The mind shares these same characteristics. An active mind is jumpy, just as we are jumpy when we are anxious. Stress churns the mind so our internal waters are choppy and difficult to navigate. When unmotivated, depressed, or afraid, the mind is inactive and, just like a dark sea, it is hard to see clearly what is really happening beneath the surface. A balanced mind—quiet, pure, and insightful—is evident in a relaxed person. The waves of the mind have been stilled. In this peaceful state it is easy to see clearly through the internal waters to the depths; we may understand what lies beneath the surface and, observing the depths of our psyches, connect to our higher selves. In this awareness of spirit we understand the limited nature of material objects and learn how to remain free from suffering. What helps still the waves of your mind? Is it a walk in nature, painting, listening to music, having a bath? Bringing balance to your overactive or inactive consciousness gives you clarity and ease.

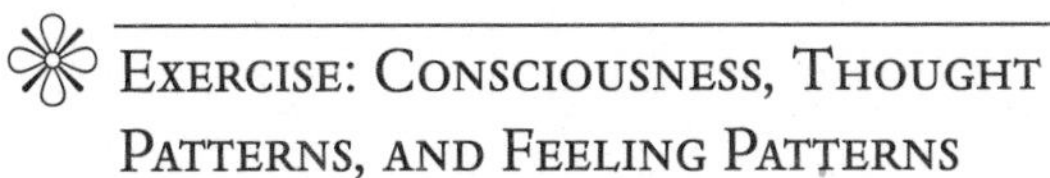

Exercise: Consciousness, Thought Patterns, and Feeling Patterns

Our physiology is directly linked to our states of mind. In order to transform or eliminate stress, we must understand how we are creating it. In the beginning, developing awareness of tension and relaxation in your body is like going into uncharted territory. We're not usually taught subtle body awareness and it takes practice to begin noticing how your body works and feels at any given moment. With time, you'll start to recognize when you are holding tension in your neck, shoulders, jaw, belly, or lower back, and you will try to avoid postures or activities that make your muscles tense. You can relax your body by simply taking a deep breath, releasing tension in the shoulders, or sitting up straight. With many years of practice, you will become greatly attuned into the workings of your whole being, including the internal organs and systems of the body, the connection between the emotions and body, and the flow of breath and energy. This exercise is designed to awaken you to the power you have over your internal environment.

1. Set a small timer to ring periodically throughout an entire day. When the timer rings, hear the last thought that was in your mind and jot it down, then practice a quick body scan by noticing what is happening throughout your body from feet to head or vice versa. Record physical observations occurring at the same time as the thought. Do not judge what you are thinking or what is happening in your body, simply observe. (Each response to the timer should only take a minute.)
2. At the end of the day, review your notes. Were different thoughts associated with different reactions in the body? List some relationships you noticed, such as: "When I thought about my teenager, my throat was tight," "I noticed my mind was on my paperwork a lot and there always seemed to be stiffness in my back," "My mind was on my morning walk and my chest felt clear." You may choose to repeat this practice over many days in order to further realize the role of your mental habits on your overall state of well-being.

Suffering Is Optional

It is often said that pain in life is inevitable but suffering is optional. This means that our beliefs about painful situations can cause a great deal of suffering (*dukkha*). The main problem in our thoughts is resistance to pain or stress, which breeds suffering. One of our yoga teachers has a story about a summer day when she was young. While splashing in a lake with her friends, she sliced her foot on the sharp edge of a clamshell. As she was sitting on the dock, crying and rinsing off the blood, one of the attending parents came over and said, "You cut your foot, but you are okay. You know it is going to hurt for a while; why be upset about that?" She understood: it didn't make sense to keeping crying over a hurt she couldn't change. She accepted the pain and it was no longer so aggressive. Once the bandage was on, she jumped back in the lake and continued splashing.

It is possible to face life's pain in the same way. Although our adult pains may be more profound than a cut on the foot, we already understand that pain such as death, crime, job loss, breakups, and so on are a part of life and also happen to be outside our control. By accepting our lives as they are, our minds relax and we are open to facing what is before us with courage and peace. Introspection and psychological awareness are the first steps in removing stress. Accepting the beliefs we find within ourselves immediately eases the suffering. We can unwind the stories we tell ourselves about the situation and instead focus on the present moment as it is. As we become more sensitive to discerning the higher self and limiting our anxieties, the last step of reprogramming beliefs is beyond conscious control; it makes itself known through calm responses and shifts in thoughts, feelings, and behaviors over time. Through yoga, our physical, energetic, and emotional responses to stress relax and we are better able to face all situations from the calm perspective of the higher self. Even the most enlightened people feel pain, but they no longer suffer with it.

Asha suffered from such a deep anxiety that it became frightening to even leave the house. Asha's Comprehensive Yoga Therapist helped her explore the beliefs underlying the fears, while teaching yoga relaxation techniques for body, breath, and mind, just as we do in this book. Progress is measured by incremental successes: walking around the block twice per week, making eye contact and saying hello to at least one stranger per day, and at least three times each day exhaling slowly while imaging anxiety blowing away. In order to meet these goals, Asha was forced to challenge the belief that it was not safe to leave the house and confront her perceptions about being unlikeable. Through small, daily adjustments, these flawed perceptions and beliefs dissipated, leaving an open curiosity about the world and others in it. As consciousness shifted, Asha became less ego-centered and approached life from the balanced perspective of the higher self.

In the olden days, when stress was not so prevalent, we were not separated from our childhood supports. One of the reasons our culture has so much stress is that we are separated from our families, childhood memories, and friends by distance and our habit of electronic connection, which is not a true connection. Having moved away and with life being so busy, we have to make special efforts to relate to those from our past, who are familiar with us and have witnessed us grow. Being with people who have known us our whole lives gives a feeling of being grounded, supported, and at ease. When we spend time with people who know us well, we see the true, higher self shine through and feel self-reliant in maintaining that confidence. The goals and intentions are your own but remember to seek assistance when required. Get community support as much as possible. Self-reliance thrives in knowing your intention, sharing it with supportive people, and acting on it.

Exercise: Small Daily Adjustments

For this exercise, in order to free yourself from anxiety, cultivate a pure, balanced intention for everyday life. Just as Asha chose to walk around the block, say hello to strangers, and make eye contact, you can make strides each day that take up little or no extra time. By holding a spiritual intention such as peacefulness, compassion, or self-love, you will experience its impression upon your states of mind, body, and breath. You may hold the same intention for months or change each day, depending on what is relevant for your well-being.

1. Without thinking too much about any of the items, spend the next 30 seconds writing down all the stressors you can. It's okay if you repeat some of the anxieties or worries—just write.
2. Pick one item from the list that you are ready to change, write it on a new piece of paper, and throw the old list in the recycle bin. Spend the next 30 seconds writing out actions and feelings that are the *opposite* of that stress. Again, don't think too much about it, just record whatever comes to mind.
3. Now, review these opposite actions and feelings and choose one that you feel confident you can accomplish. This step can be done in one of two ways: either set a small, simple goal like Asha did (more on effective goal-setting later) or commit to an intention of feeding yourself an uplifting feeling. This latter intentional perspective can be carried through everything you do if you remain aware of it.

A new, intentional perspective helps us deal with stress and transform our attitudes toward daily tasks and interactions. On the flip side, pure goals and intentions reveal contrasting attitudes within us. When we hold an intention for kindness, our unkind thoughts and actions contrast starkly, even when directed solely toward ourselves. This intentionality gives us pause; we can reflect on the source of the unkindness or other pain, learn to take responsibility, and become who we want to be. In this peaceful space, a life informed by goals of regular yoga practice or specific moments of personal awareness offers a fuller sense of self and facilitates the greatest healing. The following exercise teaches you to use your goal or intentional perspective to relax.

Exercise: Consciousness in Yoga Postures

You now know that the mind-body complex relates back and forth: our thoughts affect our brains, hormones, and nervous systems, and stress in our bodies can make us feel anxious.

Yoga postures help balance these systems and calm the mind. The benefits of yoga postures are amplified when we approach them with intentionality. Bring your goal or intention from the previous exercise to mind as you practice the following postures. If your mind wanders, refocus on your body, breath, and intention or goal.

1. Move through the following sequence, guided by your pure intention. Follow the instructions for the postures carefully and trust the wisdom of your body. Mild discomfort is normal, but the postures should never hurt. Care for yourself by approaching the postures slowly and staying present with what is happening inside you.
2. The following sequence is designed to offer you a sense of groundedness, strength, and relaxation with your personal goal or intention.

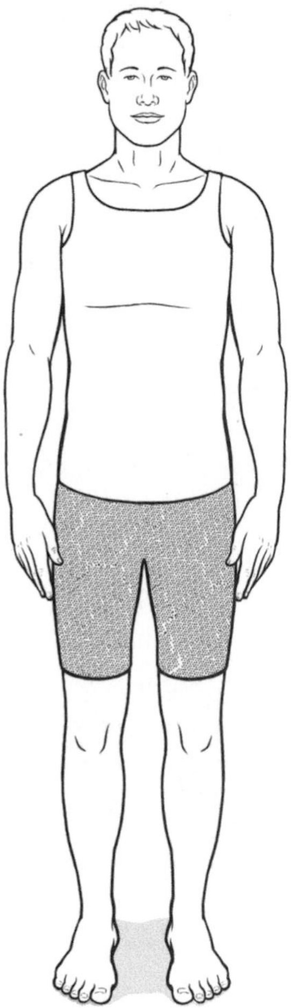

Figure 3.1
a. *Tadasana* (Mountain Pose) with Equal Breathing

Stand on the three prongs of each foot (under the big and little toes, and the heel), arches lifting away from the floor. Stack your ankles, knees, hips, waist, ribcage, shoulders, and earlobes in alignment. Keep your belly strong but loose enough to allow full, deep breaths. Feel your body surrendering to the ground and lifting skyward, relaxing shoulders, face, and breath. Stabilize yourself, connecting to a sense of being sturdy and grounded, tall and strong, like a mountain.

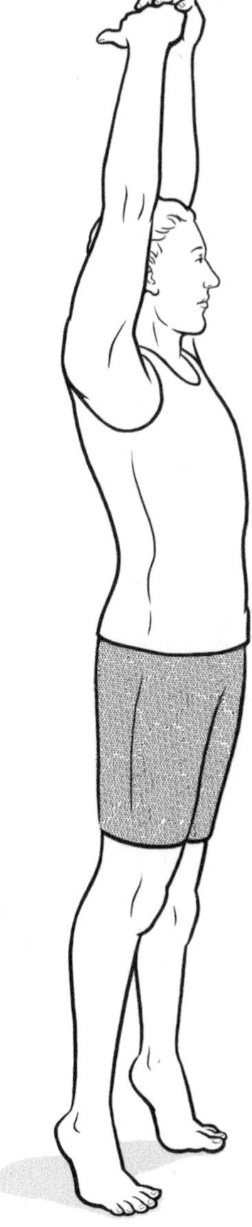

Figure 3.2
b. *Talasana* (Palm Tree Pose)

On an inhale, begin to raise your arms overhead while rolling your weight to the balls of the feet. At the top of the inhale, you will have risen to tiptoes with both arms above you, fingers interlaced and shoulders in neutral. Hold the posture for a comfortable length of time, breathing deeply, then exhale and lower your arms and heels with slow control.

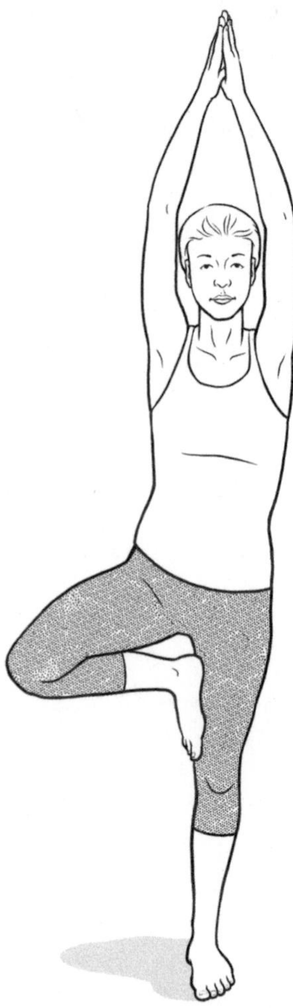

Figure 3.3
c. *Vrkasana* (Tree Pose). Repeat on the other side.

Root your left foot into the earth, envisioning energetic roots growing just as a tree's do. Plant the sole of your right foot on the side of your left leg (above or below the knee but not against it), right knee pointing to the side. The weight-bearing leg is straight, but the knee is not locked. Keep your eyes open and your gaze soft. Your palms may come together at the heart center, your arms may open overhead in a V, or you can interlace your fingers as your arms raise overhead, pointing index fingers to the sky and crossing the thumbs. Feel perfectly balanced between earth and sky, rooted into the support of the ground.

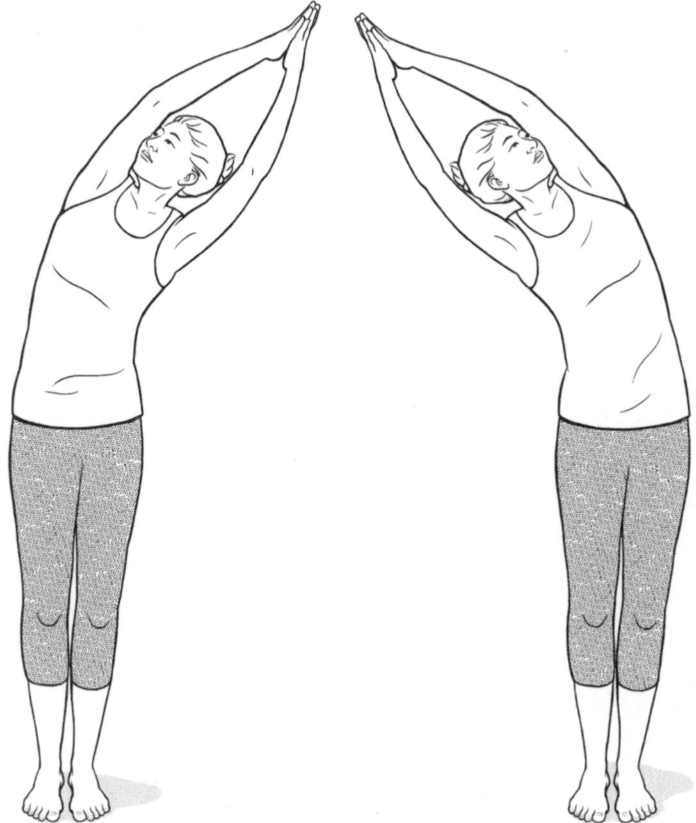

Figure 3.4
d. *Ardha Chandrasana* **(Half-Moon Pose)**[1]

Inhale your arms overhead, palms together, fingers interlaced, and index fingers pointing. Exhale, leaning your body to the right while keeping your top shoulder rolled open. An advanced option is to secure the abdominals and slide your hips to the left to increase the side bend. Make sure that your weight presses

1. This may not be the typical half-moon pose you are familiar with, which extends the bottom hand down to the floor and the top leg up.

evenly onto both feet. Breathe into ribcage, waist, and hip areas. Inhale center, exhale other side.

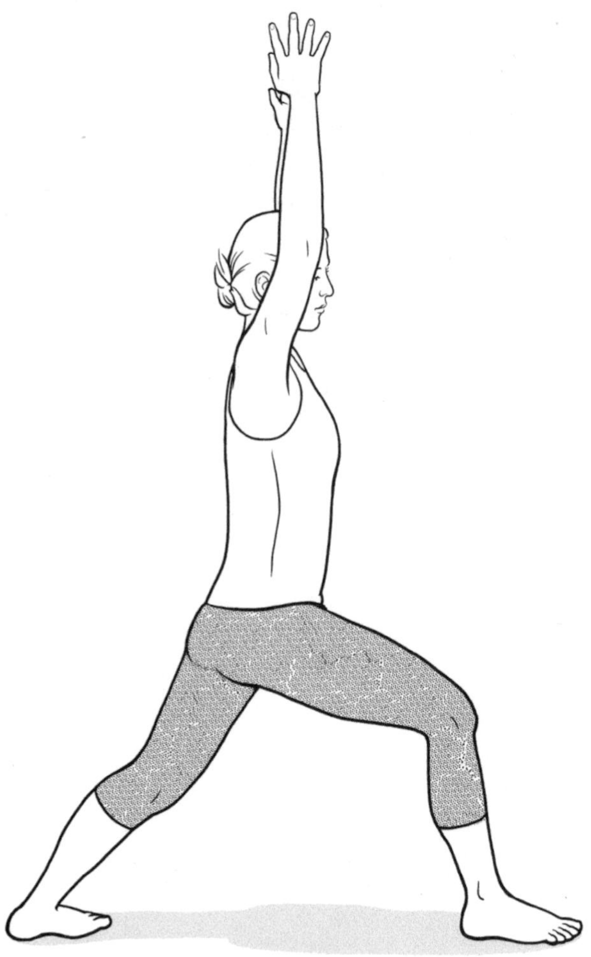

Figure 3.5
e. *Virabhadrasana I* (Warrior Pose I)

From Mountain Pose (*Tadasana*), inhale your arms overhead. Step your left leg back, turning toes out and planting through outer edge of foot into toes. Bend front (right) leg. Do not push knee past toes. Breathe strength from the earth. Repeat on other side.

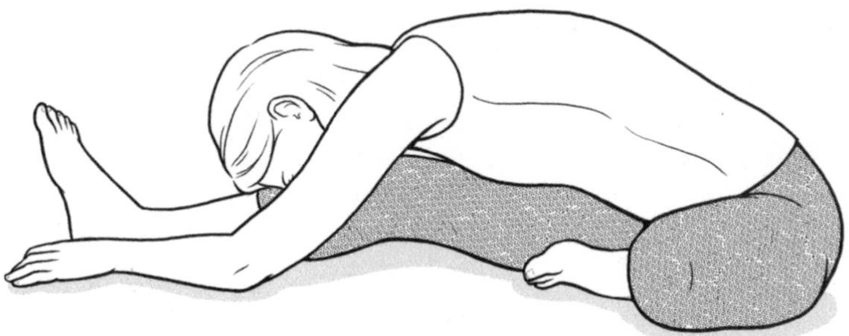

Figure 3.6
f. *Ardha Paschimottanasana* (Half Seated Forward Bend)

Bend one knee to the side, placing the sole of the foot against the opposite thigh, and bend as shown above. Repeat on the other side. If hip or back pain precludes the bend, that leg may be straightened slightly out of the way so the focus remains on one leg at a time.

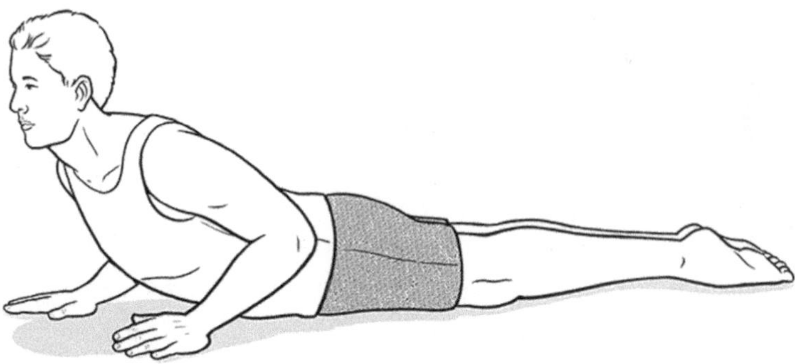

Figure 3.7
g. *Bhujangasana* (Cobra Pose)

Rest on your abdomen, palms under shoulders, forehead to mat. On an inhale, roll forehead, nose, chin, and each vertebra off the mat to a comfortable height. Open the chest by drawing the shoulders down and back. Bring strength into the lower belly and buttocks. Press into the top of the feet and pubic bone.

Feel equal intensity in lower and upper back. If breath becomes short, strained, or irregular, or if your face begins to flush, it is best to come out of the pose immediately. Repeat if appropriate. Unroll through chin, nose, and forehead, and rest on your belly with feet wide apart and toes pointing outward.

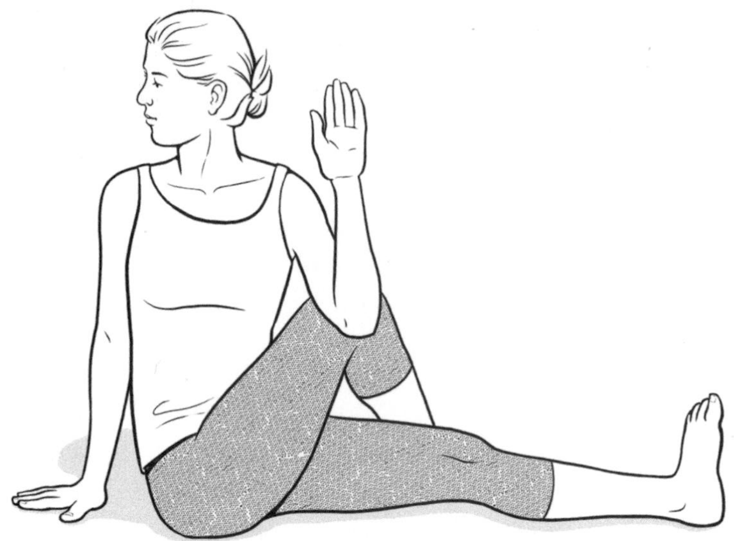

Figure 3.8
h. *Ardha Matsyendrasana* **(Seated Twist Pose). Repeat on the other side.**

From a seated position, legs out in front, bring your right leg over your left knee. Your left arm hugs the knee across your body or the outside of your left elbow presses the outside of your right knee. Rest your right arm on the floor behind you and twist around to the right, from base of spine to top of head. Look over your shoulder, keeping chin parallel to the floor and not leaning forward or back. On each inhale, lengthen your spine and relax your forehead more and more. Do not push or pull with your arms to force the twist. For a gentler variation, sit cross-legged or soles together and allow one hand to rest behind and one in front.

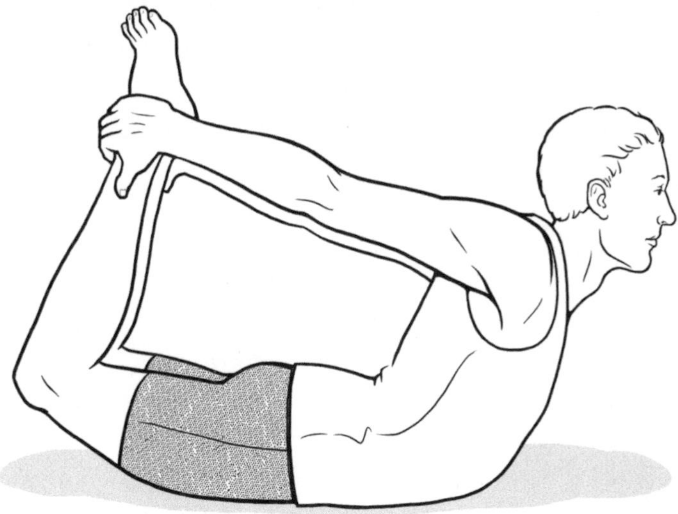

Figure 3.9
i. *Dhanurasana* **(Bow Pose)**

Lie on your belly with your hands alongside your torso, palms up. (You may lie on a folded blanket to pad the front of your torso and legs.) Exhale and bend your knees, bringing your heels as close as you can to your buttocks. Reach back with your hands and take hold of your ankles. (If they are too far away, just reach your hands back as if to hold them or use a strap to bridge the gap.) Inhale your heels away from your seat while lifting your thighs away from the floor. Roll your face, collarbones, and chest up as well, keeping your thighs high behind you and abdomen strong. As you breathe, your torso will rock on the floor. Keep knees in line with hips, neck long (shoulders away from earlobes), and gaze forward. Exhale to unroll. You may repeat the pose.

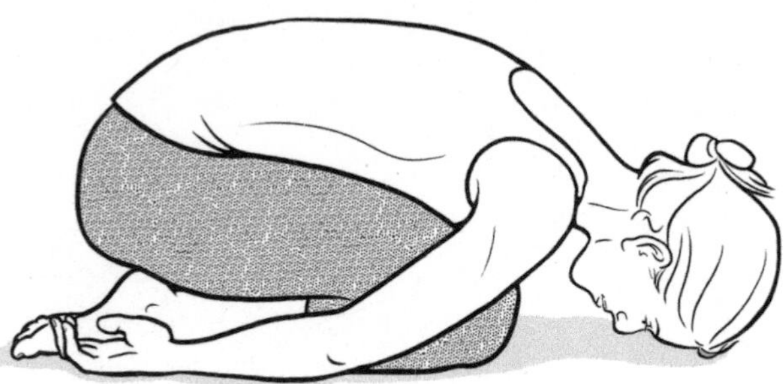

Figure 3.10
j. *Balasana* (**Child's Pose**)

Place your crown or forehead on the floor, easing your seat to your heels. Extend arms overhead or rest palms up beside your feet. You can stack your fists to make a pillow for your forehead if the floor is too far away. Breathe your wandering thoughts through your forehead into the earth. Feel your breath moving in the back of your body, stretching and healing the lungs while relaxing and energizing the nervous system.

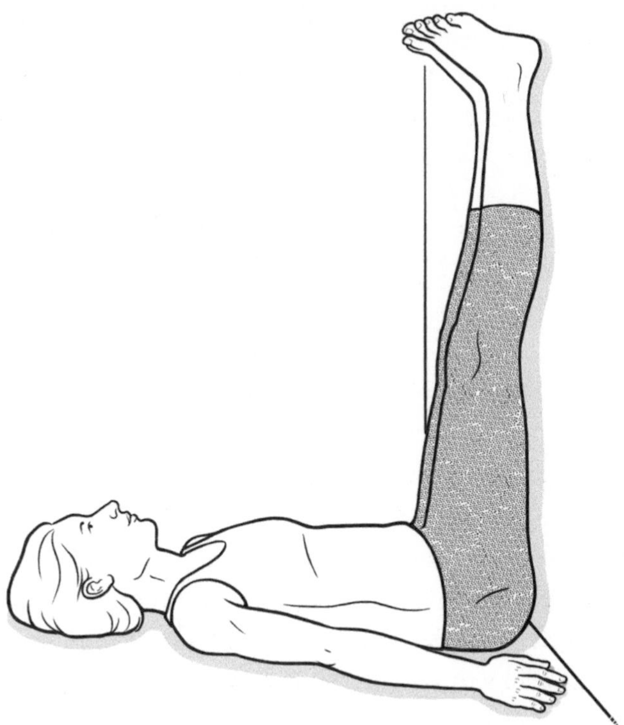

Figure 3.11
k. *Viparita Karani* **(Inverted Action)**

Rest on your back and float all four limbs into the air, allowing them to rest into their sockets. This is relaxed—no reaching or extending upward. If precautions are present, try raising one limb at a time, alternating sides, or only arms then only legs. For a more restful experience, rest your arms alongside your body and rest your heels against a wall or on a chair.

Exercise: Letting Go Relaxation

Enjoy an opportunity to lie down and call to mind your pure intention. Relaxation is an important part of yoga and is essential in removing stress and anxiety. Taking time to consciously relax the mind and body balances the nervous system and sets an internal tone of freedom from stress. This exercise gives you practice in letting go of stresses and replacing them with your goal or intention.

1. Settle yourself into a comfortable relaxation posture. Remind your muscles that they don't need to do any work right now. No matter how much they relax, the ground will hold up your body; the muscles don't have to. Melt into the earth and surrender to her support.
2. You may notice that some parts of the body hold on to the stress. Which parts let go easily? Can they help the holding places release as well? Imagine relaxation and release spreading through any tightness or resistance.
3. Begin to imagine your brain sinking into the earth as well, falling away from the front of your forehead. Neural activity moves from the frontal lobe to the mid-brain, where the action of meditation lives. All cares and worries are gone.
4. Draw in an awareness of the intention you set in the previous exercise. You may imagine yourself carrying out the goal, in your mind's eye seeing yourself feeling happy, relaxed, and accomplished. Bask in the good feeling that following your intention will bring. If any worries come up, breathe them out and bring your mind back to the image or feeling of your personal goal. Allow the mind and body to remain in this state of relaxation, basking in the feeling of your intention. Notice that holding a pure intention helps disentangle from the physical body. You can decrease the ego's grip on reality and

transform old beliefs, drifting into a quiet relaxation guided by spiritual intention.

Now that you have worked through this chapter, you may already notice that your beliefs have shifted! Harmful beliefs, such as disliking change, fearing the unknown, or wanting much of one thing and none of another, cause suffering, stress, and anxiety. Whenever we attach our sense of happiness to external or material things we suffer. It is okay to enjoy what life offers, just don't look to it for peace of mind; the ever-changing external cannot provide this. If we rely on the higher self and a pure intention to support us, all of life becomes an opportunity for yoga practice. By getting in touch with the higher self, we shift our beliefs about the world and our place in it. We will build on the power of beliefs in Chapter 6. For now, remember that, with practice, old beliefs about stress diminish in the face of connection with the higher self. Internal alignment brings harmony with the external reality.

Chapter Summary

1. The conscious mind does not know everything. It is the unknowing of what is truly within that makes us vulnerable.
2. Life is neutral; the human mind interprets the positives and negatives.
3. By understanding habitual belief patterns that lead to certain reactions, the mind is able to reshape its responses and thereby reduce or eliminate stressful reactions.
4. Know where tension is in your body so that you may relax it, in turn helping the mind relax.
5. Pain is inevitable in life; suffering is one interpretation of pain. Hence, we can limit our suffering—thereby stress and anxiety—through self-awareness.

6. Yoga practices offer the mind stillness, which leads to self-understanding and a reduction of stress. The goal is to learn about one's self during the yoga practices.

Now that you have explored your deeply held beliefs, we'll move on to examining how you care for yourself. In the following chapter you will discover how your stress and anxiety affect many levels of your being and what you can do to unwind those harmful impacts.

Chapter 4

How Anxiety Influences the Many Body Layers *(Koshas)*

To round out Part I, we are now teaching you to look at yourself as a whole being. Where Chapter 1 gave you an introduction to the process of yoga therapy for anxiety and stress, and Chapters 2 and 3 enquired into the depths of your mind, this chapter demonstrates how anxiety affects the five layers of your being (body, life energy/breath, mind/feelings, intellect, and spirit/higher self). Yoga philosophy views the whole person on many levels, each influencing the others. Stress and anxiety disturb our layers, and this chapter offers recommendations for creating ease on all layers.

The Five Layers of a Person

You are probably familiar with the idea of body-mind-spirit. Yoga expands this concept a little more, viewing the human being on five layers (*koshas*) from the body to the spirit/higher self. In addition to body, mind, and spirit, these five layers include life energy/breath (*prana*) and distinguish the lower mind from the discerning intellect. The five layers are 1) body, 2) life energy/breath, 3) mind (feelings and lower thoughts), 4) intellect (wisdom and discernment), and 5) spirit/higher self. Each of these layers exists within the next, like a collapsed telescope, moving from the obvious to the subtle. The layer of the body holds within it the life energy or breath. In yoga tradition, we are taught that breath contains life energy, the subtle animating force (*prana*). Within the breath is the mind. In this case, the mind means what we take in through the senses, including feelings, and how the personality interprets that information. The intellect is quieter and can be likened to the wise, witness self. It is the part of us that is able to discern between the ego's reactions and the reality of the higher self. The most subtle of these layers is the ineffable spirit—that still, abiding bliss of the higher self that lives within us all.

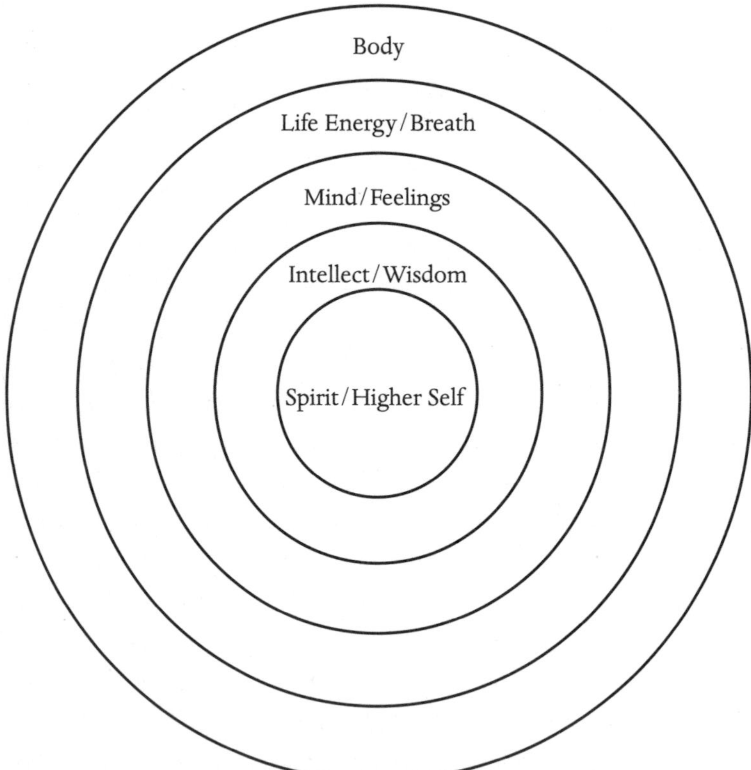

Figure 4.1: Koshas/Layers

The ancient Sanskrit text the *Upanishads* discusses human beings in terms of these five layers. The layers reveal that each level of our being is guided by a subtler counterpart. The outermost layer is made up of matter, the physical body. The physical body changes significantly over time as we age. We come to realize that we are more than just a body. Within the physical layer, and slightly more subtle, is the breath or life energy. The body affects the breath and the breath can affect the body. By developing conscious breathing practices, we influence this subtle relationship; this is the fundamental reason breathing is such a powerful component of yoga practice. When we breathe deeply into the diaphragm, the body relaxes and releases stress; when breathing is rapid and shallow, the body and mind become tense.

Within the life energy layer, and even more subtle, are our sense perceptions and emotional responses to external situations, which is the layer of the mind. When we are frightened, we gasp for breath or stop breathing altogether and the body becomes rigid or quakes. When we cry heavily, breath comes in short spurts and the body quivers. When we are content, the breath is deep and slow and the body is relaxed. These heightened states of mind have profound effects on breathing, in turn affecting the physical body. Even more subtle than the mind is the intellect. This is the discerning self, not mere intellectual prowess. The layer of intellect is the voice of wisdom that says, "Yes, I'm feeling anxious now but this too shall pass." When we are connected to wisdom through the intellect, the breath is more likely to be peaceful regardless of external circumstances. Finally, the most subtle of all the layers is spirit/higher self, the bliss layer. This is the state of universal consciousness through which we are connected to all beings.

As you consider your journey through healing anxiety, remember to perceive all five layers of yourself. By moving your perception from the obvious to the subtle, you will gradually refine your internal climate and allow the subtler aspects of yourself to inform your perceptions of and reactions to the ever-changing external world. You will also begin to focus more on nurturing your whole self. Self-care practices will involve a greater spiritual connection and can draw upon the subtle bliss that is each of our natures.

The following section reviews people on the basis of each of these five layers. As you read the various case study examples you will notice each of these different people was affected more by one layer than another. The body layer relates to movement and the breath to life energy (breath and life force are sometimes thought of as synonyms). The mind relates to the senses and emotions, and the intellect to thought patterns and reason.

Pay close attention to the areas that seem most relevant to your growth and follow those areas with more detail. In other words, if you have already practiced a lot of breathing exercises so that your regular breath is deep, but your emotions are up and down, continue doing the breathing that you already know and use your journal to work through the emotional exercises. If you treat your body very well but have trouble connecting to your inner wisdom, pass over the physical exercises of this book and continue whatever physical practice you already have, then focus your energy on exercises for the intellect. This way, the number of exercises in the book does not overwhelm you. It is most beneficial to focus on strengthening your weaker layers.

Exercise: Exploring the Five Layers

The purpose of the exercise is to get you thinking about yourself on each of the five layers. As you compare the reactions of your body, life energy/breath, mind/feelings, intellect, and spirit/higher self, you may notice some layers actually respond well to stress. You will also notice which layer tends to succumb to stress and anxiety. Awareness of your patterns enables you to shift them.

1. As a means of thinking about yourself in a general way, draw a big circle on a page of your journal and divide it into five sections: Body, Life Energy, Mind, Intellect, and Spirit. We are using this to help you discern which layer of yourself needs more attention.
2. In each of the five categories of life, describe how anxiety shows itself in or impacts that area. Consider what you have noticed about your physical tensions and other sensations, depth and speed of breath, energy levels, thoughts, emotions,

fears, beliefs, and sense of connection to who you really are when in stressful situations. You may reflect on previous exercises in this book which have helped you clarify your internal patterns.

3. Notice which layers require the most attention and which layers are already somewhat resilient to anxiety. By understanding your patterned strength and weaknesses you are able to draw upon the strengths of particular layers to support the layers that tend to weaken in the face of stress. For now, it is enough to have that awareness.

Body: Sidney's Story of Reprogramming the Nervous System Through Movement

The layer of the body includes our whole physical self: skin, organs, nerves, blood, lymph, muscles, bones, and so on. Anxiety often arises due to the constant firing of the sympathetic nervous system (SNS). When we live in a constant state of stress, the body resets its baseline to one of heightened alert: *fear.* If we are moderately frightened all the time, when something truly stressful happens, there is nowhere for our stressed nerves to go except into full-blown panic. Simple yoga postures can help calm or "downregulate" the nervous system so that over time it clears the anxiety and resets itself to a more relaxed level of everyday functioning. Yoga practices still that constant effort of the sympathetic nervous system and allows its counterpart, the parasympathetic nervous system (PNS), to bring in its calming influence. This balance between the SNS and the PNS resets the body to a healthier baseline. Movement can be a great way to do this.

Many people when they hear the word "movement" think of exercise. Some people find that exercise raises heart rate and anxiety. All kinds of unpleasant images of exercise develop in their mind. Other people might love exercise, but they tend to push hard to reach a personal best, or they exercise because it will improve their health. There is a sense of "I must exercise" and within that a feeling of not enjoying the exercise, so they follow an instructor or exercise while watching TV. These people exercise but do not pay attention to the internal signals of the body. Instead they continue to focus outside of themselves and can't wait to finish their exercises so that they can go on being "productive." In either case, movement and exercise are associated with some kind of stress.

For many people, however, movement leads to decreased anxiety by combining it with breathing, good posture, and pleasure. The chosen movement gives an internal sense of our bodies while increasing our physical capacities. This kind of exercise gives us enjoyable focus on the present moment and the movement. For movement to decrease anxiety it needs to be within our capability, combined with breathing, and pleasurable. It is not to be associated with "have to" or experienced as just "exercise." More and more research seems to indicate that regular movement throughout the day is much healthier than "exercise" once per day. The research also suggests that the activity needs to be mindful in order to decrease anxiety. Mindful movement changes the brain. Mindful movements do not necessarily have to be slow, but we have to pay attention to the sensations of the body. Tuning into the body holds us in the present, not the future where anxiety lives. The following story shares how one yoga student applied these principles.

Sidney often felt out of control, disconnected from the body, and helpless. It was recommended to practice the same five simple yoga postures every day, which are described in an exercise in Chapter 1: Stick Pose, Bridge Pose, Restorative Forward Bend, Supine Half-Moon Pose, Reclined Half-Twist Pose. The quietude of these yoga postures imbued themselves into Sidney's consciousness so that when a sense of control slipped away, the body-memory of the postures brought reconnection and groundedness. This physical presence assuaged the dizziness and racing, helpless thoughts that accompanied Sidney's anxiety. By practicing yoga poses, the nervous system began to dial back the fear response and dial up relaxation. Sidney even applied gestures of the postures throughout the day—raising arms overhead, arching the back, or folding, side bending, and twisting in a chair at work, in the washroom, even standing in line!—and this maintained a sense of calm.

Exercise: Moving Away from Anxiety

Let movement be a tool to soothe your anxiety. If you already attend yoga classes or have some form of home practice, you can refer to those for this exercise. If you are new to yoga, you may consult the Yoga Posture Table of Contents in the front of this book to help you. The purpose of this exercise is to give you a reference of personally meaningful yoga postures. This empowers you to turn to a beneficial movement practice whenever you wish!

1. Find at least one yoga posture that calms you. Bending forward or twisting the body can quiet the nervous system. You may also benefit from balance poses like Tree or Palm Tree, which help you focus, or back-bending postures like Cobra or Locust, which promote courage.
2. In an easily accessible section of your journal, start a list of postures from this and other books, your yoga classes, DVDs, or reputable online sources that relate to your anxiety in a healing way. Trust your feelings: if you enjoy the posture or it seems to soothe you, add it to the list! Continue building the list over time and do some postures from it whenever you want to calm yourself or feel like moving.
3. Consult this list in times of need and offer yourself just one of the movements in order to step away from anxiety.

Life Energy/Breath: Kai's Story of Reprogramming the Nervous System Through Breath

The life energy layer is sometimes thought of as the breath and sometimes as the animating force carried within the breath. This layer is more subtle than the body layer as we cannot actually see the breath, though we can feel it moving. Whenever we concentrate on the rhythm of our breath we are connected to the present moment. Focusing on the present rather than dwelling on the past or fretting about the future is relaxing to the mind and emotions. If we have time to sit and breathe quietly, it is likely that external circumstances in those moments are stress-free. This grounding, calming effect makes slow, conscious breathing the most commonly used technique in crisis counseling. From a yoga perspective, the life energy / breath layer is between the layer of the body and the layer of the mind, thereby serving as a bridge between the two. A deep, steady pace of the breath is relaxing to the body and balancing to the mind.

Stress impacts the sympathetic nervous system (SNS) or "fight, flight, or freeze" response. This is an adaptive response if you are being chased by a bear but is not a healthy reaction to heavy traffic or belittling comments. When the SNS is highly active, we experience increased heart rate and breathing, which transports the stress hormones and neurotransmitters through the body more quickly. This is sometimes called an adrenaline rush and includes cortisol, endorphins, and other chemicals to help the body respond to acute stress. Circulation is directed away from the digestive organs into the muscles to promote power and speed. Thoughts race and memories are encoded as sensory impressions such as random colors, sounds, and smells, rather than a linear story. The only part of the nervous system most of us can consciously control is the breath. Rapid shallow breathing tends to activate the SNS, while slow deep breathing tends to activate its counterpart, the parasympathetic nervous system (PNS). We might not be able to direct circulation or the release of certain chemicals, but we can take a deep breath, which activates the PNS, which in turn slows the heart, sends a relaxing message to the nerves, dissipates the stress-related hormones, channels blood flow back to the digestive organs, and so on. The deep, steady breathing of yoga—and in turn its activation of the PNS, is one of the reasons why yoga is a powerful de-stressor. The following story shows how a former yoga therapy client mastered anxiety by controlling the breath.

Kai lived most days in a great deal of fear. If something was forgotten at the grocery store or a phone call came at an inconvenient time, Kai would suffer panic attacks. It felt like something awful was always about to happen. A yoga therapist recommended that Kai take a deep breath every day upon waking and before every meal. This simple deep breathing practice felt so nice that Kai linked it to every red traffic light, ringing phone, or beeping timer. With each deep breath came a sense of calm possibility, as if any stress could be managed. The panic attacks became fewer and farther between as Kai's deep breaths offered a continual reminder of physiological and emotional calm. Taking deep breaths throughout the day helped Kai face life.

Exercise: Breathing Through Anxiety

This exercise teaches you the basic three-part yogic breathing. All three portions of the lungs are involved in this kind of respiration: the lower, middle, and upper lungs. When practicing breathing into each of these parts of the lungs, be sure to inhale and exhale for an equal length of time. With practice, the number of seconds breathed into each area will increase. This smooth, equal breath helps balance the mind and calm the emotions.

1. Diaphragmatic breathing utilizes the lower lungs. Sit in a tall, symmetrical, comfortable position either on the floor or in a chair. Simply place one hand on the abdomen and the other on the chest. With each inhale, feel the belly rise as the diaphragm curves downward and lower lobes of the lungs inflate. Endeavor to keep the chest still. Exhale and feel the belly deflate as the diaphragm curves back under the ribs and the lower lobes empty.
2. Now begin the intercostals, or ribcage breath. The intercostal muscles lie between the ribs and are usually so unused they tend to "lock" and prevent conscious control. When we breathe into the ribcage, it should not lift toward the chest or move the shoulders. Instead, breathe laterally into the ribcage so that you feel an accordion-like expansion into your sides and back. Spread your fingers over the lower portion of the ribcage so you can feel the sides and back. Inhale to this area, stretching the muscles between the ribs (intercostals). Your hands

will slowly move away from each other as the ribcage expands front, side, and back but not lifting up toward the chest. To exhale, relax around the ribs and let your hands come back together like an accordion collapsing. This may be the most difficult part of the three-part breath to learn as it is challenging to isolate this region. At first, you may try slouching to prevent the ribs from lifting.

3. The third step is clavicle, or collarbones, breathing which isolates the set of muscles that controls the upper lungs. Many people with rapid, shallow, anxious breath only breathe into this area of the lungs! That is not healthy; however, chest-breathing is still an important part of a deep, three-part breath when used slowly and deliberately. Place one hand on the upper chest between the collarbones. Inhale slowly, filling only the upper lobes of the lungs, feeling the upper chest expand. You should be able to feel the top of the lungs, near the base of the throat, completely fill as the upper chest rises. Release the breath, breathing out a few seconds longer than you think possible so that the upper chest is slightly concave. It may help to cough gently to expel the air in order to round the chest in.
4. Now, practice each of the three parts of the breathing process described above in a coordinated, fluid manner. Enjoy a deep, rhythmic breath. Inhale first into the base of the lungs, expanding the diaphragm, then fill the ribcage to the sides, finishing with the upper chest near the collarbones. Without pausing, exhale from the chest, then intercostals, and finish by pulling the navel in as the diaphragm expels the entirety of the breath. Breathe in and out for the same count, beginning with 6 seconds, and gradually add 1 second at a time to prolong the count, up to 15 seconds, as you practice over time.
5. Once the equal, rhythmic breath is achieved, begin to concentrate on a smooth transition from inhalation to exhalation and vice versa. Although it may be somewhat frightening at

times, avoid the tendency to start each exchange quickly. Usually, we breathe in too quickly for the first few seconds from a desire to get the air in; likewise, when beginning to exhale there is a tendency to expel the air forcefully at the beginning. Instead, attempt to breathe to the best of your capability in a smooth, even fashion.

Mind/Feelings: River's Story of Reprogramming the Nervous System Through the Senses

The layer of the mind encompasses our senses, feelings, and fleeting thoughts and impressions. In modern times, our minds are very cluttered because our lives are full of information, busyness, and powered technology. Nowadays, most people in affluent countries can simply turn on a tap when we want water, adjust the thermostat for comfort, or click some computer keys to find the answer to a question. Some of these conveniences are not necessary for healthy living, but over time the conveniences become the norm. Not so long ago, only a few homes had air conditioning and none had computers. Not so long before that, people were pumping water from wells or drawing it from the river, chopping wood to heat their homes, and growing or raising all of their own food. Ironically, there was less talk of "stress" in those less convenient times.

We are readily aware of the benefits of technological advancement; however, each new gadget also plays into both the illusion of external control and a greater sense of immediacy in all things. These factors imbue our everyday decisions with a greater sense of pressure. With that in mind, ask yourself how often you "unplug" from the world and go without electronic devices such as Internet, television, cell phones, music players, and so on. Stimuli from the natural environment is quieter and less intrusive. It is also more relaxing and helps connect us to a greater reality.

Our technology pings and dings as soon as it's time for an appointment or we have a new email or Facebook update. We just can't stop looking at our phones and are constantly interrupted. Whether we call that sensory sensitivity, ADHD, or use any other new diagnostic name, it does change the brain. This neurological change is especially true for the generation that has grown up with the Internet and smartphones. We might wonder why it is so hard to focus on a task when we sit in a classroom or in a silent environment, but we can sit and focus forever in front of the computer. One of the reasons is that in the classroom the brain does not get frequent "rewards." In front of the computer playing a game the brain gets its rewards much more frequently. The reward is a small squirt of dopamine.

Dopamine is a neurotransmitter that brings us a sense of pleasure. It makes us feel good and accomplished. The more frequently we get the dopamine squirt the more likely we are to continue what we are doing. Creators of computer games know this. They also know that the games must move fast—and so do most blockbuster movie directors, TV executives, and radio DJs. The pace of things combined with the dopamine rewards make it more difficult for us to complete tasks that take longer or do not provide frequent rewards. Therefore, we have more and more people being diagnosed with sensory sensitivity and ADHD. On the one hand, the brain is overstimulated and craves silence and peace; on the other hand, it is accustomed to the dopamine rewards. This sets up an internal conflict when we unplug. If technology is available, the brain's trained response to the dopamine usually triumphs over the need for silence.

Considering this neurological tug-of-war, it is no wonder some people have a difficult time meditating or practicing yoga that focuses on the internal senses or slowing down. The dopamine-addicted person likes the "power" yoga styles much better. In a faster-paced class they feel like they are accomplishing something the entire time and they get their little dopamine rewards. However, this quest for dopamine, no matter how unconscious, traps us in a neurological state of arousal, where beginning to quiet our stress and anxiety actually feels disquieting and nervous.

Yoga exercises for the senses have both external and internal aspects. The external aspects come in from the outside world: what is seen, heard, felt, smelled, tasted. The internal aspects involve the mind's interpretation of the sensory input. Why did it taste that way to me? What aspect of the sound stood out? How did I color the information with my past experiences? What is my brain function contributing to my version of this experience? Each of us has a unique set of reasons why we interpret sensory information the way we do.

River was very sensitive to the external environment. Easily startled by loud noises, River was constantly distracted by what else was going on and was especially aware of potential dangers. This sensitivity led to sleep issues and nervousness, as well as a lack of focus and productivity. It was a downward spiral of ever-increasing stress. As part of a yoga teacher training course, River learned yoga techniques such as focusing on a single sound and looking at a candle flame to master the senses. These yoga practices steady the mind and help create distance from what may be happening in the external world. To River, life began to seem less busy, scary, and distracting. By attuning to the higher self and witnessing the internal world rather than overvaluing what was happening on the outside, River is no longer dragged through life by the whims of the senses.

Exercise: Sensory Self-Care Strategies

Each of the five senses can be a vehicle for soothing the nervous system and reducing anxiety and stress. The following exercise cultivates a calming relationship between the inner and outer worlds via the senses. Many of us are very visual. When we remember things, we recall the imagery associated with the feelings and circumstances. Some people recall sounds more easily or bodily sensations. No matter the internal habits, the senses create a strong link between the inner and outer worlds.

1. List three calming experiences for each sense: sights, sounds, textures, aromas, and flavors that soothe you.
2. Select one of these and spend the next few minutes absorbing your awareness in that sensation. You may close your eyes and hold a flower or fresh cooking herb close to your nose. You may listen to a bird outside your window or your favorite instrument in a piece of music. You may stroke your pet or rest in a warm bath. Whatever you choose, allow your awareness to focus on that sense for 5 minutes.

3. Now that you have engaged a single sense for a prolonged period of time, notice the effect on your sense of relaxation and connection to the higher self.

Exercise: Visualization for Relaxation

1. Recall an experience that soothes your senses, such as listening to birds, watching rolling waves, or feeling a light breeze blow over your skin. As you rest in a relaxing position, begin to imagine yourself experiencing that particular sight, sound, aroma, taste, or feeling. Allow this inner experience to calm you.
2. Notice the experience of relaxing as you focus on a single sensory experience. By feeding your mind these pleasing sights, sounds, smells, tastes, and touches, the nervous system responds as if you were really in that situation. Notice the effect on your body, breath, feelings, thoughts, and sense of connection to your higher self.

Mind/Feelings: Alex's Story of Reprogramming the Nervous System Through the Mind

Physical feelings often relate to emotional states, and both exist at the layer of the mind. Whenever we avoid our emotional experiences, we are suppressing our feelings. We may avoid emotions through escapist habits, complaining, or denying individual feelings until they blend into one big mass of anxiety. As the avoidance pattern builds, years of unresolved emotions are stored in the psyche, awaiting their chance to be released. Each time a stressor or uncomfortable situation arises, these stored past emotions surface, seeking their chance to express themselves after all this time. Anxiety is not just about the present moment, but all other emotional experiences that we have not dealt with. By listening to emotions on a daily basis, we can understand the roots of anxiety and release it through gentle practices.

We are able to manage our feelings once we are ready to accept responsibility for them. Yoga psychology views emotions as reactions to life and messages about how to obtain deeper peace with the present circumstances. Emotions tell us about ourselves, and each emotion deserves respect and acknowledgement (which does not mean dwelling on it!). This idea of accepting all emotions may be opposed to a belief pattern that there are "good" and "bad" emotions. Consider that we may view passing emotions without attaching a judgment. When we are afraid of uncomfortable emotions, we become anxious about the emotions themselves! When we realize that emotions are merely a source of information, we can face them and use the information fearlessly to create better lives.

Alex suffered from anxiety since high school. Every day seemed to loom ominous with lists, tasks, and potential failures; these worrisome feelings repeated themselves well into adulthood. Alex's yoga teacher often recommended that students repeat the relaxation from class every night at bedtime for a better sleep. Alex enjoyed that feeling of relaxation in class so much that it was worth a try at home, where Alex did a simple foot to head body scan and imagined each part filling with a loving calm. Sleep began to improve after the very first attempt. Not only that, but the anxiety grew progressively better each day, as well. When stresses cropped up during the day or fearful emotions began to build, Alex remembered the loving, calming cues from the relaxation and became peaceful.

Exercise: Body Scan Relaxation

You can use this practice as a baseline experience to see how your body feels and what level of relaxation is present. You may apply autosuggestion techniques at any time to remind your body to relax if it is holding tension. With regular practice of the body scan, you will learn to retrieve all kinds of emotional feedback from your physical self.

1. Find a comfortable position: sitting with the head supported, reclined slightly, or lying down.

2. Remain in this position practicing for up to 10 minutes; any longer will often result in sleep. If you do doze off, your body likely needs more sleep and you might want to consider going to bed earlier or scheduling naps.
3. Start to slowly "scan" your body from the crown of your head to the soles of your feet (or feet to head), all the while observing a slow breath. This scanning can best be described as bringing full awareness to whatever part of the body you are paying attention to. In so doing, the feeling and sensations in those areas increase. Depending on the level of ease in each part of your body, this scan will clue you in to which muscles or joints are at ease and where tension may be hiding.
4. Continue to be a witness to your body, creating some distance by changing "my" to "the." For example, instead of saying "my shoulders are tense," say "the shoulders are tense." This small change in language simply acknowledges the existence of tension while removing you from the direct experience of it—in other words, you are no longer labeling yourself as the tension! You have more space to objectively observe the body and keep the mind aligned with the higher self. As the lungs exhale and release air, the neck releases; then the back releases and so forth. This language creates a more detached perspective that greatly assists in relaxation.
5. When you have scanned the whole body, pause for a moment or two to integrate. If you are not feeling drowsy, you may repeat the scan up to two more times. See if you can allow the tense parts to relax a bit more on each subsequent scan. Your potential for relaxation is amazing!
6. In time, you may use this practice to also witness the emotions that pass through the mind, the way clouds pass through the sky, changing shape and moving on. Similarly, thought patterns can be witnessed in this neutral fashion. Train yourself to become an objective observer by learning to activate the relaxation response.

Intellect: Morgan's Story of Reprogramming the Nervous System Through the Intellect

When we consider the layers of a person, it is simple to distinguish the body from the breath. Separating the mind from the intellect is more subtle. The intellect is the layer of discernment, wisdom, and higher thought. Think of it this way: the mind is of the senses and includes our *feelings*—both what we feel through the sense of touch and our emotional feelings. Emotionally based lower thoughts belong to the mental layer as well. The intellect is closer to the spirit and is in the realm of ideas. Intellect helps us relate to that higher self and discerns between the material world and ultimate reality, or the lower self and the higher self.

Based on this theory of the layers of a person, we are able to call on the intellect to guide the mind toward more spiritual feelings. Remember, when we think of the layers of a person, the intellect offers acumen; it is about wisdom, not about intelligence level. An ancient yogic writing, the *Katha Upanishad*, describes the relationship between the layers, where the layer of the higher self is the revered owner of the chariot, while the layer of the body is the mechanical vehicle. The spiritual wisdom of the intellect steers the chariot by holding the reins of the mind. Thus, we are instructed to use our intellectual wisdom to direct lower, more fearful parts of the self. By following our higher quest for self-realization, the layer of intellect discerns between that which is peaceful and that which is fearful. The intellect steers emotional contents and thoughts—the layer of mind—in the direction of that peaceful higher self.

Autosuggestion from the Voice of the Intellect

You have likely heard of some benefits of hypnosis (these do not include clucking like a chicken or other comedic suggestions!). Hypnosis is a psychological technique used to tap into what lies beneath conscious awareness and create a shift from there. Experts in hypnosis have created audios you can purchase, of varying quality. Self-hypnosis is the process of using conscious thoughts to reprogram the not-conscious material. This practice of personal reprogramming is found in many traditional yoga techniques, usually referred to as autosuggestion. Autosuggestion, or suggestions made to oneself, harnesses the mind and intellect to promote spiritual alignment. Common examples of autosuggestion techniques include affirmation, positive self-programming, self-hypnosis, body scan relaxation, and visualization.

It is the role of the intellect to discern between the ever-changing lower self and our true, spiritual nature. No matter how much we practice, most of us have some weaknesses in our personalities; stress is a common example. We may intellectually understand and comprehend the meaning of relaxation, but remain unable to connect with it in daily life. When you work with autosuggestion, bring your awareness to any personally harmful tendencies you discover. These tendencies have their roots in beliefs that are stored beyond your conscious awareness. These beliefs are often irrational and arise from early painful experiences. The intellect can unearth these old beliefs and purify them, thereby connecting you more deeply to your higher self and spirit. The next exercise aims at transcending the not-conscious, anxiety-causing attitudes and connecting with the truth of the higher self.

During the last ten to fifteen years our ability to look into the brain has improved. We use various technologies to see what happens in our brains when we meditate, reflect, observe, or receive sensory information. We can even see how our brains change when we change our thinking. All these studies have altered our belief that the brain cannot modify or develop after a certain age. We now know that the brain never stops developing, as long as we introduce mindfulness and variety into our thinking and activities. Mindfulness and variety create new pathways in the brain. Then again, if we don't change our thinking and activities, the old pathways get stronger. If we keep thinking and doing the same things, the results of these thoughts and actions will also be the same—not only in our external lives but internally as well! We will respond to stress in the same way, and our anxieties will be the same.

Awareness activities such as meditation, mindfulness, autosuggestion, and attentive movements can be seen as a way to begin something different in the brain: a newness or an interruption of our usual way of thinking and being. This introduces a change in the brain. Indeed, studies have revealed that the introduction of meditation and awareness practices shows positive changes for anxiety. By incorporating such activities and remaining the conscious director of our thoughts, the areas of the brain that fire during worried thinking, anxiety, and even pain responses begin to alter!

After years of suffering from panic attacks and chronic nervousness, Morgan was diagnosed with an anxiety disorder and prescribed medication. Although the pills helped, it was not the final solution. Morgan continued looking for ways of reducing the ever-present anxiety and enrolled in a year-long yoga teacher training program to study the practices and benefits more deeply. Morgan began to think of life in different terms, separating the ego's state of anxiety from a subtler, underlying state of continuous freedom. By discerning what to focus on, such as the breath, nature, or compassion for others, and when to apply various yoga practices such as deep breathing, yoga postures, or autosuggestion, Morgan soon weaned from the medication and realized a freedom from anxiety like never before. Although this may not be everyone's experience, it is a testament to the power of the wise intellect when yoga is applied to someone's life.

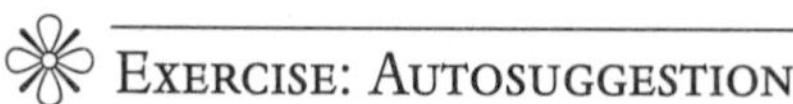

Exercise: Autosuggestion

A simple way to harness the power of the intellect is through directed suggestion. The discerning layer of intellect can speak to the other, busier layers and calm them. This exercise will help reprogram not-conscious beliefs, as well as the baseline nervous system functions related to them. When used in conjunction with yoga postures, breathing exercises, and self-care strategies, autosuggestion can alter our entire internal climate.

1. Begin in a comfortable relaxation posture; take a few deep breaths and begin to witness your inner experiences, accepting the thoughts, emotions, and sensations that pass through your awareness. Acknowledge that the part of you doing the witnessing is a relaxed and objective observer to your inner world. At first it may be challenging to connect to that witness self and that is okay; just do your best.

2. From that objective witness place, begin to offer suggestions to relax. As with the previous body scan relaxation, you may begin at your head or your feet and name the body parts in order as you suggest that they relax, pausing after each area to notice the effects the suggestion has.
3. A sample of cues are:

   "I am relaxing the toes, feet, and ankles ... I am relaxing the calves, shins, and knees ... I am relaxing the front and back of thighs, the hips, seat, and pelvis ... I am relaxing abdomen and lower back ... I am relaxing middle back and upper back ... I am relaxing the chest ... I am relaxing the fingers, hands, and wrists ... I am relaxing lower arms, elbows, and upper arms ... I am relaxing shoulders and neck ... I am relaxing head and face ... I am relaxing eyes, nostrils, inner ears, tongue ... I am relaxing the feelings ... I am relaxing the thoughts ... I am connected to my higher self...." Be creative and find the cues that best suit your needs to bring you into a place of deep relaxation. Notice that the layers of mind/feelings, intellect, and spirit/higher self are included in the cues.
4. Once you are comfortable with this practice, you may begin to apply more personalized affirmations: "All is well." "I am strong and stable." "Every day I am more relaxed." Select phrases that connect with you deeply—the possibilities are endless!

Spirit: Gale's Story of Connecting to the Subtle Layer of Spirit (Higher Self)

The innermost layer, spirit, or higher self, is very still and quiet. When our bodies feel lethargic, unwell, or agitated, when our breath is erratic, when the emotions are stirred up, when we are not connected to our sense of inner wisdom, it is challenging, if not impossible, to connect to the layer of the higher self (although it is always there). If you think of a time when you felt most like who you really are—calm, content, in wonder of the world—you were likely communing with your spirit/higher self. Once the mind is quiet enough to sense it, spirit/higher self can guide all of our everyday moments. The higher self can color all of our activities and interactions with peacefulness and upliftedness. When we unite the layers of ourselves, the spirit/higher self shines through all of them.

Gale was a yoga teacher who secretly struggled with anxiety. Months would go by and Gale would feel nothing but lost, talking about spirituality with students while not feeling it from within. Gale realized that although yoga was a fundamental aspect of daily life, there was no joy in it. Gale was practicing from a place of "should" and "have to," rather than listening to the authentic voice of the higher self. Gradually, Gale incorporated music into a daily practice, spending some time singing or playing instruments before meditation. This brought a sense of connection to Gale's true, higher self and every day after this self-expression there was a greater sense of possibility and wonder.

Exercise: Spiritual Fulfillment Through Your Higher Self

The following reflection exercise asks you to remember yourself before you were confined to specific roles, duties, and expectations. The secret route to your higher self is imagination. This exercise will work best if you are honest about the joy you have experienced, even if the overall tone of your childhood was not so joyful.

1. Breathe deeply and relax. Think back to when you were in kindergarten. What did you do for fun? Did you draw, color, talk with others, "play pretend," build things, or ...? Use the free-association technique of listing as many things that you enjoyed as a young child as you can in 30 seconds (it's okay to repeat yourself).

2. Repeat this process, reflecting on what you enjoyed around the age of eight years old. How did you play? What were your favorite things?
3. Repeat this one more time, reflecting on yourself at the age of twelve.
4. Read over these lists and commit to doing one thing from one of the lists in the next week. It can be as simple as picking berries or fall leaves, watching squirrels, building with blocks, scribbling, or going to a local park and playing on the swings.

It is important for each of us to find our own path to the higher self. Ultimately, all of our answers are within and we must turn to our own expertise, rather than giving our authority away to anyone else. The spirit/higher self is wise. In the next part of this book, we will examine the five different paths of yoga and help you investigate what practice most connects with your higher self.

According to yoga philosophy, we are composed of five layers. The idea of these layers of a person is familiar to you with the popular talk of body, mind, and spirit. Yoga discerns the breath out of the body-mind complex and also acknowledges the important role of the intellect as the bridge between mind and spirit/higher self. As you work with yourself on these layers, be sure to continue seeing yourself as whole person, not five separate pieces. The layers wrap around one another, similar to an onion. Anxiety affects each of the five layers and at the same time limits our awareness of them as we put too much attention on the worried mental state. An example of anxiety operating on all five layers is when stress occurs, our muscles get tense, and we lose control of the breath, feeling ever more fearful. As the emotions become more overwhelming, the thoughts race, no longer discerning a higher perspective on the situation or thinking spiritually. By connecting to the higher self and harnessing the power of your intellect, you have the power to guide yourself back to alignment with the higher self, balanced emotions, deep breath, and a relaxed body.

Chapter Summary

Even though we do not completely understand the human mind-body complex, yoga gives us a language to understand the whole person.

1. Yoga unites all facets of our lives to a higher self.
2. Each person is an individual and requires a unique approach to balance, health, and self-realization.
3. Connection to the higher self brings more confidence to life and alleviates anxiety.
4. Comprehensive Yoga Therapy tools reveal imbalances in the layers and an individual path to strengthen them.
5. Balance applies to all facets of life simultaneously.
6. Continue with practices that are already in your repertoire of self-care. This book applies yoga philosophy, breathing, postures, meditation, nutrition, relaxation/sleep, and personal attitudes to removing stress and anxiety.
7. We are composed of five layers: body, life energy/breath, mind/feelings, intellect, and spirit/higher self. Anxiety affects each of these layers and at the same time limits our awareness of them.
8. Movement, deep breathing, sensory self-care, and choosing/directing our thoughts all help bring the spiritual layer into conscious awareness.
9. When we live in a constant state of stress, the body resets its baseline to one of heightened alert via the SNS. Yoga practices still that constant effort of the SNS and allows its counterpart, the PNS, to bring in its calming influence.
10. A deep, steady pace of the breath is balancing to the mind and emotions.
11. Gadgets fortify our illusion of external control and increase our sense of immediacy, which ultimately creates pressure.

12. Each of us has a unique set of reasons why we interpret sensory information the way we do; yoga practices help calm the relationship between internal and external worlds via the senses.
13. We are able to manage our feelings once we accept responsibility for them. Emotions are a source of information and listening to them helps us understand the roots of anxiety and release it.
14. Turn to the intellect to guide the mind toward spiritual feelings and virtues and away from nervous thoughts.
15. Trust the call of your spirit or higher self. If you feel pulled to explore a healthy aspect of self-expression, go for it!

Part I of this book has given you the chance to tune in to your stress and anxiety and understand some of their root causes. You have examined your beliefs—both conscious and not-conscious—and now know yoga techniques to build your beliefs away from stress. You are able to perceive your anxiety through all layers of yourself. In Part II of this book, you have the chance to discover routes out of anxiety by following each of the five yogic paths. One path may suit your approach to life or your stress triggers more than the others. Have fun exploring the yogic paths of psychology, intellect, health, work, and relationships.

Part II: The Five Yogic Paths

In this section, you will learn about the five paths of yoga: psychology (*raja*), intellect (*jnana*), health (*tantra*), work (*karma*), and relationships (*bhakti*). Stress and anxiety arise from a sense of separation from the higher self or who we really are. Yoga offers paths of reconnection to the higher self that can be customized to each student. Yoga addresses individual differences in aptitudes, learning styles, obligations, and interests. Not all people practice yoga in the same way, yet all people will benefit from some form of practice. Traditional texts of yoga teach five paths to the higher self: one for those who practice meditation, one for those who follow the intellect, one for those who prioritize the body-mind complex, one for those who work, and one for those who love. Most of us follow all of these five paths at the same time in varying degrees. Enjoy the following chapters as you learn about which paths you are dominant in and how to balance yourself in all these areas of life.

Chapter 5

The Yogic Path of Psychology (Self-Understanding)

The eightfold path of yoga, the yogic path of psychology, is known as the "royal path" (*raja*). It is an eight-limb process of understanding the mind and becoming established in meditation, as taught in the ancient text *The Yoga Sutras of Patanjali*. By following the eightfold path, you will systematically come to understand the nature of your psychology and gain mastery over your state of mind. The eightfold path involves having an external ethical code of restraining harmful behaviors and an internal ethical code of observing purity. This path includes yoga practices of postures, breathing, sense mastery techniques, and concentration to help steady the mind so that we can see clearly into our psychology. Mental and spiritual concepts of meditation, and ultimately a pervasive sense of well-being, round out the eight limbs. The eight limbs of classical yoga offer a road map to a peaceful lifestyle. Through limiting harm, cultivating serenity, moving enough, breathing deeply, choosing uplifting feelings, and focusing the mind, we are readily able to live a calm, meaningful life. This chapter supports you in establishing a meditative lifestyle as a tool for adapting your psychology, thereby freeing yourself from stress and anxiety.

Meditation's Ultimate Goal Is Self-Understanding

Once you understand how your mind works, you can have peace. The disturbed mind is only a mind that we don't understand yet. By understanding an aspect of our mind, we accept it. You may remember having great difficulty in grade school, like being teased for poor reading skills. Perhaps the difficulty arose because you needed glasses and no one figured that out until second grade; of course reading skills were behind! Once it was understood that you couldn't see the writing on the blackboard, it made sense that the skill was amiss. Until that understanding, however, you would have felt anxious every day of grade school. You can apply this yoga psychology formula to anything:

Situation + Misunderstanding = Anxiety around the situation
Situation + Understanding = Peace of mind

Meditation teaches us about ourselves and our lives. It slows the world long enough for us to see things more clearly. The world may be seen. The mind's reactions are revealed. Perspectives will clear with time and space to understand. The ultimate teaching with meditation is no longer a goal of mind-quieting; we have come to realize it is all about *mind understanding*. The measure of a successful meditation is that you are learning about yourself. Evaluate everything in this chapter based on something that you learned about yourself. Define meditation as anything that quiets your mind and offers you a good lesson.

Yoga incorporates psychology, the study of the mind, as a part of its philosophy, in addition to relating other layers of being. It differs from modern psychology in the sense that yoga looks at the entire human being to uncover the deeper realms of reality. When psychology was first introduced as a study in the late 1800s, it examined the realms of the conscious and subconscious mind only. This has changed in recent years; presently, there are many psychological approaches that integrate the entire human being. This means that yogis understood thousands of years ago what we are only beginning to understand today: that the body, life energy/breath, mind/feelings, intellect, and spirit are intrinsically linked. In order for significant understanding to occur, one piece of the puzzle cannot be given more weight than the other. Yoga aims at a complete purification of the human being through the path of meditation. This path is outlined clearly in *The Yoga Sutras of Patanjali*, starting with eliminating negative behaviors and cultivating positive ones, moving to purifying the body and working with energy and breath, ultimately progressing toward meditative states that culminate in understanding the mind.

The Ethical Foundation of Yoga Practice

Pure psychological intention is fundamental to a *well-adjusted life*, not just to yoga practice. As you learn to cultivate intention and connect to the higher self, you'll start to do the same in your daily actions. Many of us live disconnected from our intention for doing things, whether in work, relationships, or some other area of life. How can we embody our most inspired self if we aren't clear on the reasons behind our actions?

In learning to cultivate a stress-free intention, let's consider *The Yoga Sutras*, one of the most revered Indian texts on yoga philosophy and practice. This work was compiled approximately two thousand years ago from an oral tradition that is much older. It offers the eight limbs of yoga, which provides the structural framework for a yoga life.

The Eight Limbs of Yoga
1. Restraint of negative behavior (Yama)
2. Observance of positive behavior (Niyama)
3. Yoga postures (Asana)
4. Breathing and energy (Pranayama)
5. Sensory mastery (Pratyahara)
6. Concentration (Dharana)
7. Meditation (Dhyana)
8. Enlightenment (Samadhi)

The eight limbs of yoga begin with our external behavior and progress inward to include perfect understanding of our own minds. The initial steps lay an important foundation for the more subtle practices that follow because our thoughts and behaviors are the first things that create mental stress. Following the eight limbs leads to physical, psychological, and spiritual health. It might be apt to say that yoga therapy for anxiety is about purifying the thoughts first in order to reach a calm state. And in order to slow the thoughts down, we have to understand why they are there in the first place! That's why we talk about yoga psychology as a way of understanding yourself.

For our present purposes, we're going to explore the first two limbs of the eightfold path, the restraints and observances. They outline ethical principles to help us live an orderly and harmonious life, and give direction on how to practice pure intention.

Restraining Harm

The restraints are the first limb of the eightfold path. We are advised to restrain anything that causes harm to others or *ourselves*, through action, word, and even thought. It is most challenging to restrain from harming ourselves, as so many of our thoughts create stress. Non-harm guides the other four restraints: truthfulness, non-stealing, moderation, and non-craving.

Restraints (Yamas)
Non-harm (Ahimsa)
Truthfulness (Satya)
Non-stealing (Asteya)
Moderation (Bramacharya)
Non-craving (Aparigraha)

Exercise: Cultivating Non-harm

The following brief exercise supports you in creating a non-harming, or loving, internal climate. When we remove harmful habits, especially mental ones, we leave ourselves open to a more peaceful inner world. Stress and anxiety are rooted in harm. Contemplate the following and allow this first precept of yoga psychology to amplify your sense of peace.

1. Consider which of these restraints relate to your stress and anxiety right now: non-harm, truthfulness, non-stealing, moderation, non-craving. Remember to think of these on as subtle a level as possible. For example, you likely don't steal things from stores, but you may steal joy from yourself by

worrying about the future. You may not tell lies, but anxiety often arises from not seeing the truth of a situation. In your journal, answer the question for each of the five restraints: "How does this precept relate to my stress levels?"

2. Select the restraint that offers the greatest opportunity for positive change and remember it during each day. Do not attempt to practice all the restraints at the same time, just select one or two that are relevant to your current situation. When stress and anxiety arise, breathe deeply and contemplate what your selected restraint feels like. This shift in mental focus alone is a big step in not indulging the stress and worsening anxiety. Focusing on a restraint rather than a worry is soothing to the psyche.

Protection from Harm in Meditation

Because meditation has so many benefits, the dangers are rarely mentioned. If any unpleasant experiences occur, speak with a yoga or meditation teacher or yoga therapist. If you are not working with someone right now, see Appendix C on finding a yoga therapist. If meditation doesn't seem to be working for you, shift your practice to a mind-quieting exercise like walking, reading, journaling, or attending a yoga class. Be careful to avoid any of the common dangers mentioned below.

- **Causing more stress:** Uncomfortable feelings from the past or present may arise through the inner quiet of a meditation practice. If you worry a lot, be careful that meditation does not create an inner whirlwind where stresses or other painful feelings keep circling you.
- **Spiraling thoughts:** There may be a downward spiral of thoughts or obsessing on a single point. If you spend a lot of time alone or tend to dwell on things, meditation can be a time when those spiraling thoughts take over. Make sure that your meditation feeds peace and not any self-harming negativity or obsessive thinking.

- **Daydreaming:** Similar to a spiraling thought, daydreaming takes us away from self-understanding. If you are prone to fantasizing, be careful that this process does not unknowingly distract you from the quiet acceptance of your present life, no matter what your situation. Be where you are now.
- **Dissociation:** Removing yourself from the present moment can be a protective process, especially for a child or a victim of some abuse. Later in life, this dissociation can repeat itself, causing disturbances in less intense stressful situations. Meditation can trigger dissociation. If it does for you, change the method to something that quiets you but does not separate you from the present moment.
- **Headaches:** Headaches may arise during or after meditation because of a newfound awareness of tension that was already there. Alternatively, if the mind stays too busy during meditation it can lead to a headache. If meditation makes your head ache, begin by shifting your approach. If it continues, move on to mind-quieting activities instead.

If any of these dangers arise in your meditation practice, accept them and shift your practice. Instead of a formal meditation, other mind-quieting activities like walking, journaling, or drawing can help you slow down your thoughts and learn about yourself, which is the purpose of meditation in the first place!

Observing Purity

The second limb of the eightfold path is observance of wholesome behavior: purity, contentment, effort, self-study, and surrender to a higher reality. Along with the restraints, the observances form the foundation of spiritual practice. Where the restraints hold back negative thoughts and behaviors, the observances cultivate positive ones and are governed by purity.

Observances (Niyamas)
Purity (Saucha)
Contentment (Santosha)
Effort/Discipline (Tapas)
Self-Study (Svadhyaya)
Surrender to a Higher Reality (Ishvara Pranidhana)

Purity and stress cannot exist together. When we feel anxious, we know that we are not in a pure state. It's okay! This awareness is the first step toward purity. On a physical level we practice purity through healthy food choices, adequate water intake, regular exercise, relaxation, proper hygiene, and all those habits that help reduce stress. Purity in the mind comes from positive thinking and healthy choices about what we mentally consume, such as the television shows we watch, the music we listen to, and the company we keep. Spiritually, we engage in purity through yoga practice or through prayer, meditation, inspirational readings, and community activities. The first thing yoga psychology teaches is a balanced state of mind. Applying the restraints and observances truly limits the influence of anxiety in the body-mind complex.

Meditation has caught the attention of big schools such as Harvard and the University of Rochester, hospitals such as the Mayo Clinic, and media outlets such as the *New York Times* and the BBC. Many if not most medical schools now teach meditation, often in the form of Jon Kabat-Zinn's Mindfulness Based Stress Reduction (MBSR). The Cleveland Clinic even has a meditation app that you can download from their home page. There is plenty of evidence that meditation decreases stress and anxiety. These changes include physiological alterations such as decreased heart rate and blood pressure, improved sleep, diminished release of cortisol (a stress hormone) from the adrenal glands, and a decrease in perceived pain. Research also suggests that the reason meditation is so effective in decreasing anxiety is due to "non-physiological" changes such as looking at situations from a new angle, being more present and less reactive, and gaining a new self-understanding.

As the mind and body are purified through everyday choices, meditation becomes easier. Meditation is of great benefit to anxiety as it cultivates a sense of "witness," or being able to watch the stresses flow through the mind without becoming involved in them. Meditation also opens our minds to options. We no longer feel trapped by stressful situations, but rather, we can focus on choosing how to respond through the filter of calm purity. The locus of control shifts from the outside (the stressful thing that happened) to the inside (our chosen response). Additionally, meditation gives us some mastery over the nervous system and our physiological stress response so that we can intervene with relaxation before becoming too anxious.

Kelly, as a high-powered corporate lawyer, felt a great responsibility to do a good job of protecting large companies while at the same fulfilling responsibilities at home and connecting with the family. As the children grew, Kelly became aware that missing irretrievable moments was harming everyone involved. The teacher of corporate yoga classes at the law firm sometimes mentioned not doing harm and finding more contentment through witnessing and accepting life. Kelly contemplated these ideas while doing poses and breathing deeply throughout the day. Mental focus shifted more toward self-care, which compelled Kelly to spend more time at home. Interestingly, this actually brought *more* success into the work arena as well, even though Kelly felt less pressure there than ever before. Kelly's duties stayed the same but the state of mind, and ultimately quality of life, was transformed.

By combining the restraints and observances with movement, breathing, and mental focus, yoga philosophy seeps into all areas of life, truly supporting our state of confident calm.

Anti-Anxiety Attitudes

The third limb of the eightfold path involves the physical practices of yoga (*asana*). Again, this limb works with the others to help amplify and embody them. The restraints provide specific examples of harmful behaviors to avoid. Instead, by observing pure concepts such as peace, compassion, or courage, we can replace the self-harming state of mind with a pure state. The observances highlight healthy behaviors we can use as a focal point for physical practice. Different yoga postures carry various attitudes and work synergistically to cultivate various internal effects based on the external position.

What physical positions bring you relaxation? Immediately you may think of resting in Corpse Pose or curling up on your side or splaying onto your stomach. Broaden your perceptions now and think of the most relaxing positions other than lying down. It is important that you are comfortable while meditating, but if you lie down to meditate you will fall asleep!

Different yoga postures have different effects on the body and mind; we offer some options on the following pages.

Psychology in a yoga pose practice is known as "posture," "attitude," or "conscious mental pose." Whether you are feeling anxious, depressed, joyful, upset, or enthusiastic, the emotion is visible in the alignment and physical expression of your yoga postures. For example, if you are very stressed, you will likely continue to lift your head in forward bends instead of relaxing the neck, while a depressed person will slump right over, usually with laziness in the legs. A joyful or confident person will be long through the spine while a fearful student contracts. In short, our attitude reflects our state of mind, and our position in a yoga posture reflects our attitude. What body position or habit reflects your stressed-out attitude? How about your attitude of relaxation?

Exercise: Poses and Contemplation of the Opposite Attitude

This exercise gives you the chance to explore what attitudes are revealed in your body and how you can adapt them through yoga postures and intentionality. The yogic path of psychology teaches that by selecting a particular attitude, you retrain your state of mind. Programming that mental state into the body through yoga postures amplifies the benefits and helps you integrate mental shifts more quickly.

1. Consider a current stressor or a common trigger to your anxiety. What are the underlying feelings associated with it? You may journal to understand these more deeply.

2. Do you notice if one of the restraints (non-harm, truthfulness, non-stealing, moderation, non-craving) is relevant to this situation? You can ask yourself which observance (purity, contentment, effort/discipline, self-study, surrender to a higher reality) relates to the stress.
3. As you practice the following yoga postures, focus on the attitude assigned to each posture (a chart is available below for quick reference). Notice the effects of these positions and attitudes on your sense of anxiety. Practice each posture in a steady and comfortable manner, letting go of the tension you are holding in your body and mind. (Note there is a difference between tension and strength. Some muscles will remain strong in these postures.) You may rest between each posture to fully integrate the effects. Take your time and enjoy the experimentation process. If you only have time for one or two of these postures, it is okay to practice them individually, just be sure to do so gently as you may not be warmed up and don't want to overstretch. The goal is to center yourself on a spiritual attitude and be receptive to its positive feeling.

Posture	Attitude
Talasana (Palm Tree Pose)	Reaching to the highest
Vrkasana (Tree Pose)	Grounded
Virabhadrasana II (Warrior Pose II)	Confident
Chakrasana (Wheel Pose)	Balanced
Ardha Matsyendrasana (Seated Twist Pose)	Calm and clear
Poorna Titali (Butterfly Pose)	Transformation is possible
Simhasana (Lion Pose)	Strong and courageous
Ustrasana (Camel Pose)	Fortitude
Ananda Balasana (Happy Baby Pose)	Playful, curious
Makarasana (Crocodile Pose)	Protected, quiet, relaxed

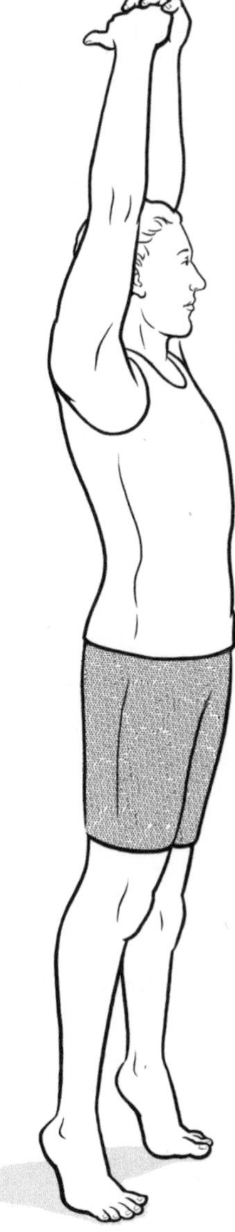

Figure 5.1
Talasana (Palm Tree Pose)—reaching to the highest

On an inhale, raise your arms overhead while rolling your weight to the balls of your feet. At the top of the inhale, you will have risen to tiptoes with both arms above you, fingers interlaced and shoulders in neutral. Hold the posture for a comfortable length of time, breathing deeply and feeling yourself reach to the highest, then exhale and lower your arms and heels down with slow control.

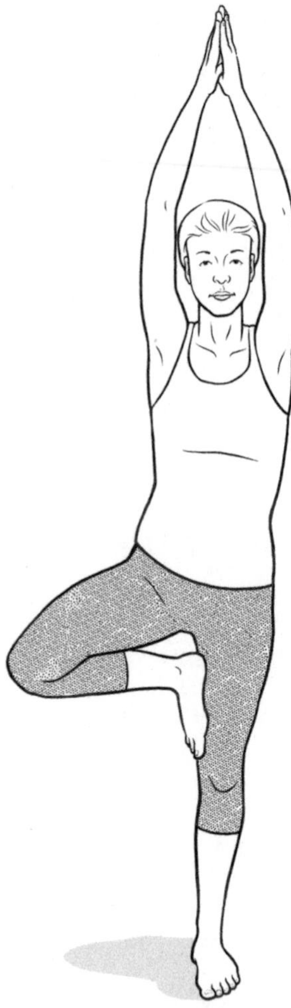

Figure 5.2
***Vrkasana* (Tree Pose)—grounded. Repeat on the other side.**

Root your left foot into the earth, envisioning energetic roots growing just as a tree's do. Plant the sole of your right foot on the side of your left leg (above or below the knee but not against it), right knee pointing to the outside. The weight-bearing leg is straight, but the knee is not locked. Palms come together at heart center. Feel rooted into the support of the ground.

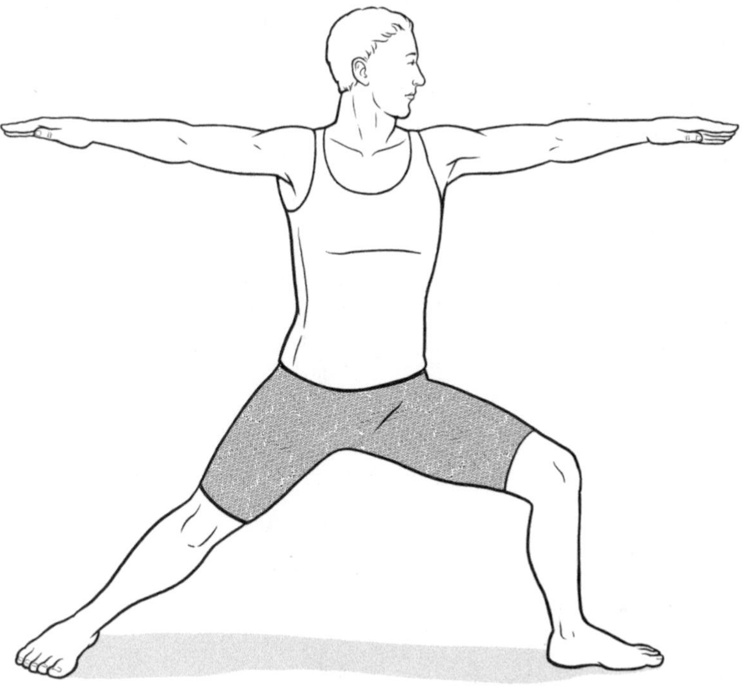

Figure 5.3
c. *Virabhadrasana II* (Warrior Pose II)—confident

Step to face the long edge of the mat, standing wide-legged. Turn the front foot to 90 degrees, toward the front short edge of the mat and the back foot slightly toward the front. Inhale and lift your arms so they are extended at shoulder height, pointing toward the front and back. Turn your head to gaze steadily past the front hand while your torso continues to face the long edge of the mat. On the next exhale bend the front knee until it is directly over its ankle. Keep the torso and hips square while shifting the weight toward the front leg and foot, pressing into the outer edges of the feet. Repeat on the other side.

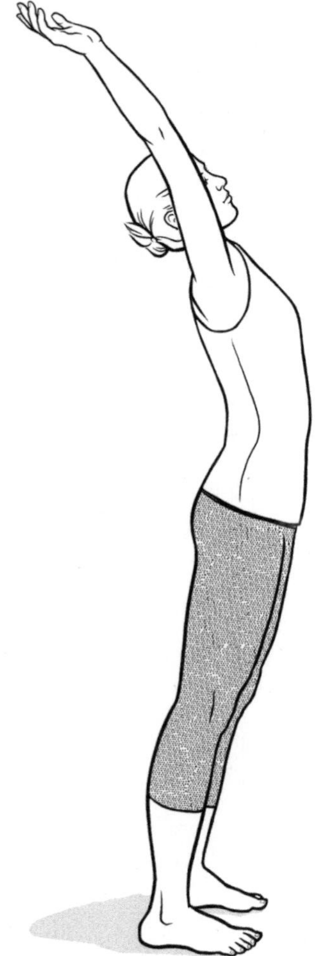

Figure 5.4a
Chakrasana a (Wheel Pose a)—balanced

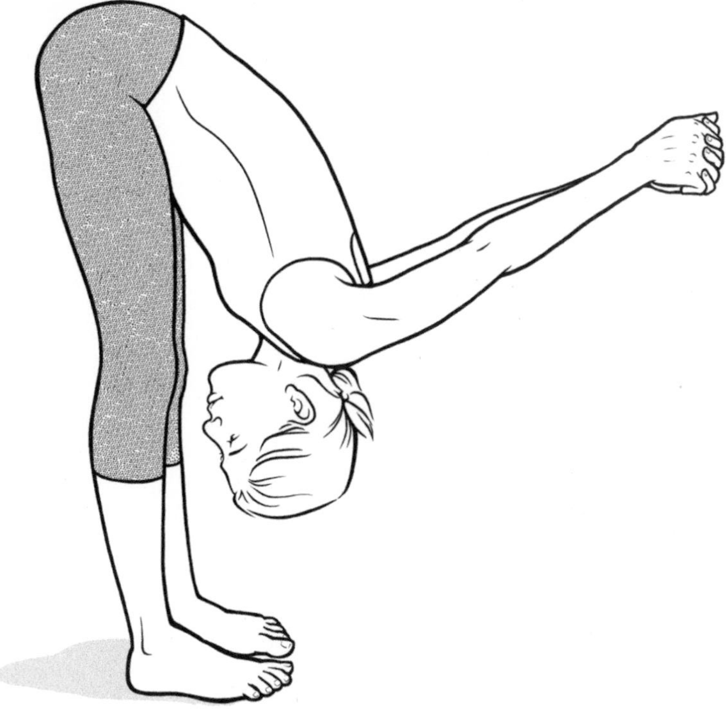

Figure 5.4b
d. *Chakrasana b* (Wheel Pose)—balanced

Step your feet back to hip-width apart. Inhale your arms overhead and feel the front of your body open forward and up as you reach your biceps beside your ears. Exhale, extending the spine long and forward (you may bend your knees slightly if you have lower back issues). Bring your arms down, around your sides, and behind you to interlace your fingers behind your back. Relax the neck, throat, and shoulders while lifting your hands and arms up. Inhale, releasing the arms down and around, and reach yourself back up to a tall, arms-overhead position. You may repeat this practice a few times, feeling the balance between front and back, up and down.

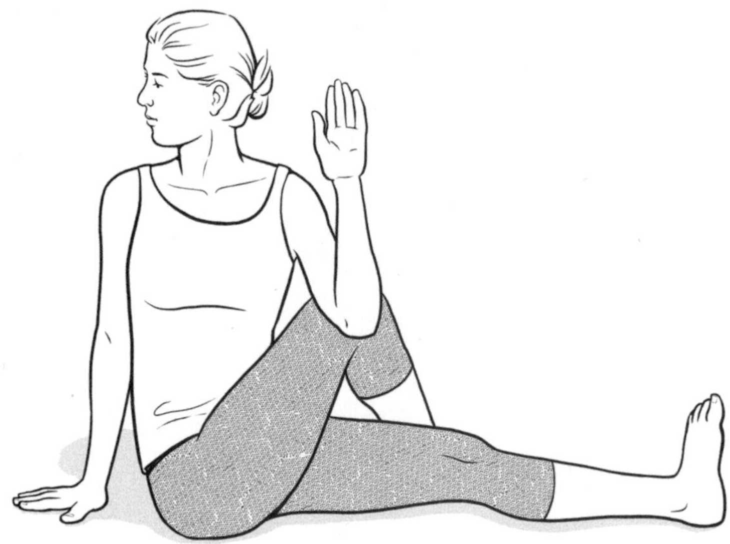

Figure 5.5
e. *Ardha Matsyendrasana* **(Seated Twist Pose)—**
calm and clear. Repeat on the other side.

From a seated position, legs straight out in front in of you, bring your right heel to the outside of your left knee. Your left arm loosely hugs the knee. Place your right hand behind your hip (do not lean back on this arm) as you twist around to the right, from base of spine to top of head and lightly. Look over the right shoulder, keeping your chin parallel to the floor and not leaning forward or back. On each inhale, lengthen your spine and relax your forehead more and more. Do not push or pull with your arms to force the twist. For a gentler variation, sit cross-legged or with both legs in front of you and allow one hand to rest behind and one in front.

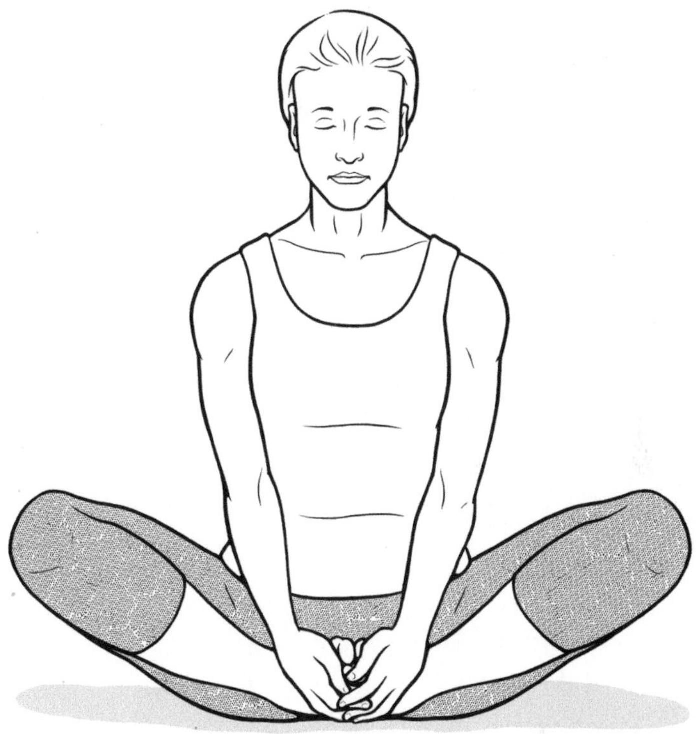

Figure 5.6
f. *Poorna Titali* (Butterfly Pose)—transformation is possible

Maintaining a tall spine (you may wish to sit on a cushion), draw the soles of your feet together, allowing your knees to fall open to each side. Hold on to your toes, feet, or shins, or, if you feel like you are tipping over backward, bring your hands behind your hips instead. You may slowly inhale your knees up and exhale them down, like butterfly wings, as you contemplate personal transformation. It is an option to fold forward in this pose.

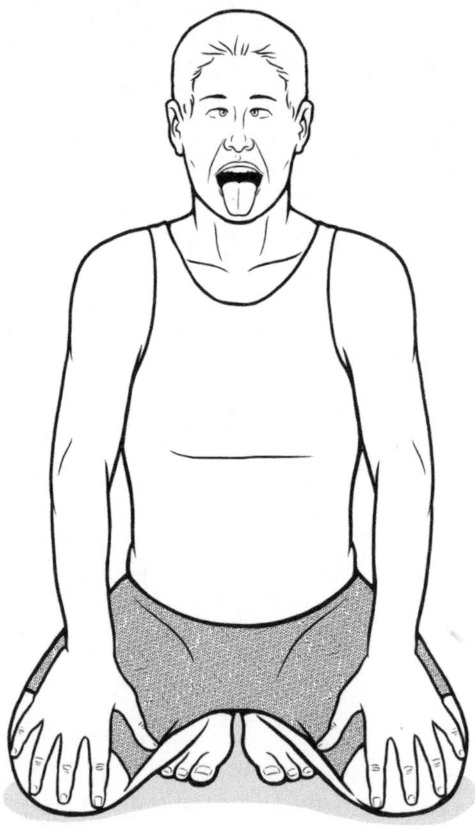

Figure 5.7
g. *Simhasana* (Lion Pose)—strong and courageous

Sit on your heels. If that is uncomfortable you may choose any seated position, including in a chair. Spread your fingers out over your knees. Stick out your tongue toward your chin as far as possible and stare upward toward the center of your forehead. Inhale deeply through the nose and exhale through the mouth, making a sound like a lion roaring. Some people will tone "Ahhhh" as if singing, while others make a breathy, toneless "Ahhhh." If you decide to truly roar, which can be cathartic, remember to project from the diaphragm in order to protect the throat. Repeat three or more times.

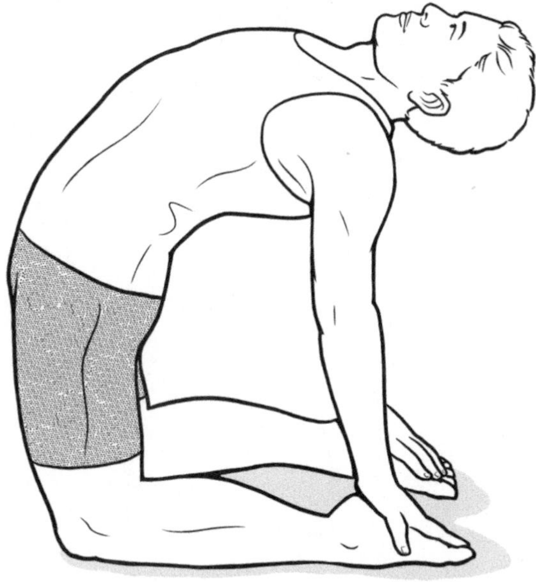

Figure 5.8
h. ***Ustrasana*** **(Camel Pose)—fortitude**

Lift the seat from the heels so you are standing on your knees, legs shoulder width apart. Place your fists on your lower back, preferably at the sacrum. Keep hips above the knees as you press the pelvis forward. Lift each of the following parts forward then up: low belly, solar plexus, heart, throat, face. If your core is strong and back very flexible, you may reach back to hold the calves or heels. Do not over extend. Exhale and reverse the actions as you come out of the posture, keeping the core strong.

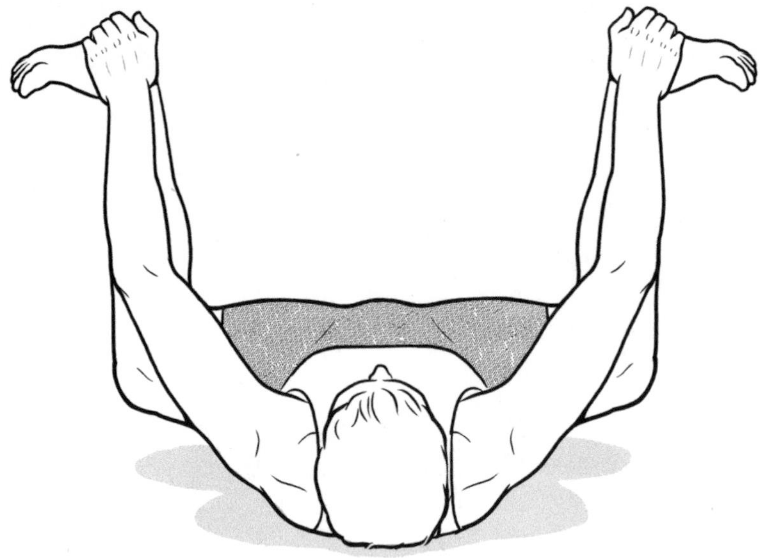

Figure 5.9
i. *Ananda Balasana* (Happy Baby Pose)—playful, curious

Lie on your back and extend your legs up into the air. Reach up to hold calves, ankles, or soles of each foot in its respective hand. Allow your knees and feet to open to the sides, drawing them toward the underarm space or beside the ribcage. Your legs will roughly make the shape of a right angle, with the shins perpendicular to the floor and the feet to the sky, not the seat. Breathe into the opening pelvis as hips, back, and neck relax. Let yourself play here!

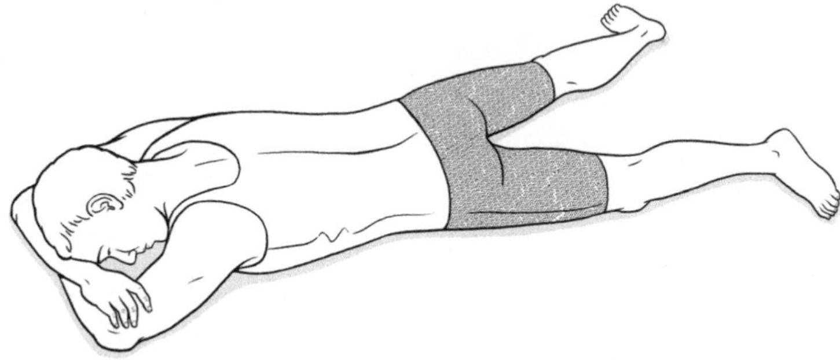

Figure 5.10
j. ***Makarasana*** **(Crocodile Pose)—protected, quiet, relaxed**

Lie down on your abdomen with your forehead or cheek resting on the back of your hands or folded arms. Bring your legs wide apart with toes facing the outside. Enjoy the diaphragmatic massage on each inhale and a complete letting go on the exhale. Feel the earth protecting your vulnerable places as breath by breath you relax. Hold this posture and quiet yourself for as long as you wish.

Exercise: Relaxation on Attitudes

These attitudes of yoga postures can be applied to a resting state as well. Holding a certain anti-anxiety attitude in yoga postures makes it active, while relaxing with that same attitude integrates it in a passive way. When we are relaxed, the psyche is open to integrating feelings, attitudes, concepts, and change on a deeper, more permanent level. This exercise is a perfect opportunity to understand more about the nature of your own mind. Enjoy the following relaxation, knowing it is helping to reprogram your psychology.

1. Choose one of the attitudes you cultivated in the previous exercise, such as grounded, balanced, calm, or playful, as a focus for relaxation. You can use this attitude as a powerful tool to release any tensions in the body. Simply lie in a comfortable

relaxation posture and begin slowly tuning into your relaxing attitude. Enjoy how its soothing feeling washes over you, fills you, and calms your body, breath, feelings, and thoughts.

2. Allow any errant thoughts, emotions, memories, and the like to flow into your relaxing attitude where they are accepted and nurtured. It is as if the attitude receives all the mental drifting and soothes it. Feel all tension being healed by the relaxing attitude.
3. Start to feel a balance in yourself on all levels. Be passive as you allow your senses to visualize, your emotions to feel, or your mind to think about the attitude. With continued practice, this relaxing feeling will become ever more familiar and gradually replace the presence of anxiety.

Anti-Anxiety Breath

Breath is the limb that follows yoga postures on the eightfold path. Anxiety is a condition of the nervous system, which responds to our psychology as well as the external environment. Breath is the only associated physiological response of the nervous system that can readily be brought under conscious control. Although yoga offers us a host of breathing techniques, it is enough to simply bring a calm mind to the breathing in order to effect a change. In other words, your psychological awareness can slow the breath. By bringing awareness to your breath, anytime, anywhere, you can begin to assuage your anxiety.

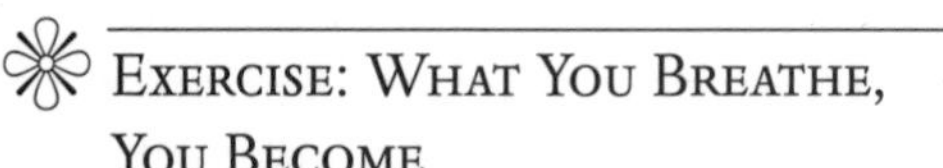

Exercise: What You Breathe, You Become

The yogic path of psychology offers a lot of simple wisdom about the workings of the mind. An important point is that whatever we focus on while breathing deeply, relaxing, or meditating becomes stronger within us. In other words, what you breathe, you become. It is wise, then, to consciously focus on what we want more of when we breathe deeply. This exercise takes you through the process of attuning your mind to your attitude, which can serve as a lovely meditation.

1. Begin a breathing exercise such as diaphragmatic breath or three-part breathing. As you relax into the rhythm, bring your attitude from the above poses and relaxation exercises to mind. Breathe your attitude.
2. As you inhale, you may use affirmations to name the attitude you are cultivating, such as "I inhale peace" or "Breathing in, I connect with courage." Uniting the breath with attitude enhances its effect on your state of mind and physiology and helps integrate it into your psychology. By using this practice, the anxiety triggers actually work to strengthen your stress management skills!

Exercise: Prolonged Exhale

The following practice regulates the nervous system and elicits a sense of ease and relaxation. It quiets the mind to prepare it for meditation. You are about to use the support and pressure of the ground to prolong the relaxing phase of breath: the exhale. Enjoy the feeling of lengthening the exhale. You may choose to incorporate your attitude into this practice, as well.

1. Lie on your stomach in *Makarasana* (Crocodile Pose) as described above. In this position, the vulnerable belly is completely protected and held by the earth. This support creates a slight resistance to each inhalation, bringing greater awareness to the breath. It also facilitates a much deeper exhalation, as the pressure of the ground encourages a full exhale, like a sigh.
2. Use that sighing effect to release tension, feeling it flow away with each exhale. These complete exhales make space for deep, revitalizing inhales.

Mastering Sensory Input

Our modern world is full of external sensory distractions: beeping phones, chiming computers, incessant traffic, idle chatter, and so on. Sense mastery (*pratyahara*) is the fifth limb of the eightfold path. It teaches the importance of withdrawing or balancing our relationship with the senses so we are not so distracted by the business of fleeting external disruptions. Anxiety can make the internal world feel equally busy, with its own realm of fears, emotions, projections, and analyses. This busyness limits meditation's ability to help us with our stress, as we find ways of distracting ourselves from becoming quiet and looking inward.

The yogic path of psychology is teaching you to discover how your mind works. Learn about how you relate to sensory input and which of your five senses seem to trigger the greatest number of errant thoughts. Stress is the main reason for most distractions. The mind tends to use the senses as an excuse to daydream about our anxieties. Conversely, a second reason for sensory distractions is that the mind uses sensory phenomenon as a reason to avoid facing the stress. This avoidance is a defense mechanism.

Let's face it, anxiety and stress are the thinker's problems. Most people with anxiety have high aptitudes and above average talent, often with a good education or strong creative leanings. Paradoxically, the intelligent are very good at figuring out reasons to worry. These sensitive people are capable of knowing the thoughts of others because they are intuitive and smart. If they weren't so smart, their anxiety wouldn't be as bad. They wouldn't know what other people were thinking. They wouldn't find so many mistakes when double-checking their work, wouldn't have so many unfulfilled ideas and dreams … you are smart enough to get the picture!

The human brain is tremendously bright so there must be a reason why people have all these anxiety-producing behaviors—from a physiological point of view, there must be some reward. While there is a psychological dimension to the underlying reasons for behavior, there is also a physiological process. The study of the brain is still in its infancy; however, we do understand that you are given a dopamine response every time you're externally validated. In other words, happy chemicals are released inside the brain when something you like or are familiar with happens on the outside. So every time you receive a text, or someone compliments you, or you see your favorite character on TV, you get a little high from the small squirt of dopamine released in the brain. Unfortunately every time you check to see if you got an email or text message and you didn't, your disappointment can lead to a sense of isolation and possibly a slight dose of depression. Your anxiety may also increase. This negative response compels you to check your computer or smart phone more frequently to get the dopamine squirt that will make you feel validated and like you belong. Thus, whenever you repeat a patterned behavior, consider that you may be doing it from anxiety.

When that moderate impulse, like texting, social media, or television, doesn't work anymore the stakes need to get higher. In order to make life feel good enough, you may seek addictions like alcohol, drugs, promiscuity, or gambling. The flipside is that the more extreme our behaviors, the more extreme the consequences and the more dire life feels their absence. What you do to get rid of your anxiety can make it worse.

This is possible even if the behavior is healthy. Remember, it is not the behavior itself but the feeling we bring to it that determines its effect on us. Two elements of lifestyle choice relate back to external validation. When we need others' approval, we seek something from the outside that gives us an internal feeling of happiness or ease. We could choose to exercise, eat right, relax, breathe deeply, and so on, but if we are expressing stress within the healthy behavior because we need external validation, then we turn what could be a healthy lifestyle choice into stress. A second aspect is taking the flawed logic that if we do something unhealthy in a healthy way it changes its effect on us. Some folks tell themselves, "If I just do my deep breathing I can text all day long" or "If I keep my spine straight then I can watch TV for hours" or "If I stretch and rest my eyes on occasion, I can troll the Internet for trivia until midnight." It doesn't work that way. We don't have the luxury of piling certain behaviors or attitudes on one side of the scale so that we can pile whatever we want on the other side. We are whole beings; thus, we undo stress by working with our entire being. A healthy lifestyle choice is coupled with *internal* validation and an attitude of *internal* peace.

Exercise: Relating Lifestyle to Anxiety

1. Does any of this discussion about the senses bridging the internal and external world resonate with you? Do you do things to help keep your anxiety at bay that eventually lead to more anxiety?
2. Journal some ways you relate your lifestyle choices to your anxiety. What external behaviors do you routinely use to soothe yourself? Some examples might be:
    - I check in with the children because I know they will say nice things to me.
    - I triple-confirm plans because I don't want to be left alone.
    - I am always late because I have to check that I haven't forgotten anything.
    - In the middle of the night my mind cycles through problems.

    There are countless other examples of ways that anxiety affects our lifestyles. List some of yours.

    While soothing the senses may seem delightful, the journey to the quietude forces us to move through, understand, and release emotional discomfort. If you are already prone to stress or anxiety, the quieting process is very difficult. Exploring the senses and understanding how we relate to the external world brings our deeper issues to the fore. When the mind is calm the pain surfaces. This is where the restraints, observances, postures, and breathing practices can help us relax through the deeper processes of unwinding the mind and learning to focus. By calling the senses away from the outer world and back to their source, we become more focused on the mind and inevitably more capable of attaining a deeper meditative state. Now the telephone can ring while we are relaxing and it is not distracting because our senses are internalized.

Even within us, we may sense distractions, discomfort, and stress. As we experience life, we generally tend to judge experiences as pleasant, unpleasant or neutral. When a pleasant sensation arises, we want more of it. When something we judge as unpleasant arises, we want to avoid it at all costs. And when something neutral arises, we hardly pay any attention to it at all. We tend to be unconscious of the pulls of greed (attachment to desires) and aversion (which can range from simple avoidance to downright hostility). We are also largely unaware of the vast range of experiences we interpret as neutral, because they simply do not command our immediate attention. Sense mastery practices train us to become aware of sensations and how we navigate life based on our relationship with them. As sense mastery practice progresses, we can more readily see how our judgments and perceptions influence each other. We become more attuned to the relationship between our mental habits and our stressful reactions to the world around us. This empowering awareness offers a pure, in-the-moment experience of life.

Exercise: Soothing the Senses

You may already be using exercises to soothe your senses without even knowing it. Listening to birds or relaxing music, gazing at a fire or candle flame, or luxuriating in a warm bath are all sensory exercises. One of the simplest things most of us do to relax the senses is look out a window or at a scenic picture. Practice the following exercise to attune to your sense mastery skills.

1. Look out the window or at a soothing picture for 1 to 3 minutes. Become aware of your eyes softening as you regard the imagery, slowing your breath, and relaxing your body.

2. Notice how this soft visual regard shifts your sensory action from groping outward. The senses relax and passively take in information from the external world, transforming it to an internal relaxation. Rather than reaching from the inside out into the world to see what we can see, the senses (in this case the eyes) relax and *receive* information. Not only does this bring greater focus, it also allows extraneous sensory information to wash over the mind without attending to it.
3. You can repeat this exercise by listening to one sound, smelling a fresh herb or fragrant flower, holding a piece of fruit in the mouth, or stroking a pet's fur. Any sensory input can be applied to this practice. The more you practice *receiving* sensory information from the outside world, rather than actively reaching for it, the more you shift to an internal frame of reference about the world around you. In time, this will leave you less affected by passing external circumstances as your inner psychology strengthens.

Meditation to Alleviate Anxiety

The final three limbs of the eightfold path are concentration (*dharana*), which is the effort to focus, meditation (*dhyana*), the pure mental state, and enlightenment (*samadhi*), which has many levels. The eight limbs of yoga differentiate between concentration and meditation. Most of what modern people "do" to meditate is actually a concentration practice. In order to concentrate, we set the mind to one object and bring it back every time it wanders away. When we are able to hold concentration for a longer period of time, there is a physiological and mental shift in state and this change in state is meditation. In meditation, brainwaves move from beta to alpha and, eventually, theta waves. Breath deepens, heart rate slows, thoughts unwind, emotions are soothed. You do not *do* anything to make this happen, just as you do not *do* sleep. The seventh limb, meditation, is a shift in consciousness brought on by prolonged practice of the sixth limb, concentration.

For this section, we combine the limbs of concentration and meditation. Technically, meditation is an altered state of consciousness that arises from prolonged concentration. Usually when people talk about meditation they are actually describing concentration. The last three limbs on the eightfold path work together like this:

- Concentration builds mental strength and ability.
- Through concentration the physiology shifts and consciousness moves into a deep, clear state of awareness.
- Prolonged awareness leads to enlightened perspectives.

Meditation is as simple as bringing complete awareness to a single subject.

Contrary to popular belief, meditation need not involve sitting perfectly still with no thoughts. Though they may not want to admit it, even those who have reached the highest states of meditation sometimes think about what's for dinner instead of their meditation. Longtime meditators still have thoughts! The last thing we want is for you to start feeling anxious about being a perfect meditator. The point of anti-stress meditation is just to learn something about how your mind works. You don't have to be enlightened or purely still and blank within yourself. If each time you sit and concentrate you are able to glean insight, that is a good meditation!

For example, after a particularly stressful day Blair sat down to meditate, hoping to work out the emotional tension and enjoy an evening outside of work. Instead, Blair repeatedly wondered about supper: what the protein would be, which veggies were in season, the local farmer got a new dog. Again and again Blair's mind would drift to supper then wander away on a daydreamy tangent. At the end of the meditation session, still frustrated, Blair wondered, "Why did I think about what's for supper? Why was I so interested in the vegetables and the farmer?" Blair realized that due to the busy day, there had been no lunch break at all. Also, because of special projects, Blair had gotten out of the routine of daily walks in the ravine at the farm. Realizing these seemingly small shifts in habit had completely overtaken the meditation practice demonstrated their importance. From then on, Blair was careful to find some time to eat during the workday, no matter how busy, and to spend time in nature despite the demands of career. Enquiring about the meditation process, no matter what the "results" of the practice were, makes the meditation successful. The goal of meditation for stress and anxiety is to simply slow things down relative to where you are right now. The yogic path of psychology teaches that any amount of time dedicated to quieting and understanding the mind is time well spent.

The path of meditation can be divided into two streams: awareness, or active meditation, and concentration, or seated meditation. The awareness branch of meditation observes every moment of passing reality through wholehearted presence. The concentration branch, on the other hand, is a seated style of focusing the mind on one subject and ignores all other stimuli. There are five types of concentration meditation: breathing, visualization, mantra, prayer, and contemplative inquiry.

Exercise: Meditation for Your Type

Instructions for meditation are simple, but the practice itself may not be easy! As discussed above, meditation may not be best for very anxious people because the mind will use the time to worry. Ironically, meditation is one of the best tools to alleviate anxiety once other calming routines are in place. Awareness practice is recommended to help reduce stress, as awareness can be brought to any situation. Simply by bringing full attention to a situation, we are cultivating an awareness meditation. This helps us calm ourselves by being more aware of the breath, our thought patterns, and our options for responding, rather than reacting, to the situation. The following exercise gives you a chance to explore which of the meditation types steadies your mind most easily.

Because meditation can trigger more worries, we recommend performing each of these practices for only 1 minute in order to clearly observe the effect they have on you. Gradually, you may increase to 90 seconds, then 2 minutes, and so on. Perform each of these sitting in a tall, dignified, and relaxed position with eyes closed or cast downward. You may notice that the minute passes quickly for some of the techniques and seems to drag for others. This is a clue to which type comes most naturally to you. Time flies when you're having fun!

1. **Breathing**: Follow the breath. When the mind wanders, refocus on the breath. After 1 minute, you may journal your observations.
2. **Visualization**: Imagine a soothing snapshot, such as a scene in nature. Focus on the beauty of this still image. After 1 minute, you may journal your observations.
3. **Mantra**: Select a word or short phrase and repeat it slowly to yourself. After 1 minute, you may journal your observations.
4. **Prayer**: Think of something you deeply appreciate, such as music, art, or growing food in a garden. Offer gratitude to wherever it is this creative miracle comes from. If you already have a prayer practice, use that instead for the next minute. After 1 minute, journal your observations.
5. **Contemplative inquiry**: Contemplate the life of someone you admire. This can be a religious figure, personal hero, or a vision of your future self. Prayer is another way to practice this type of meditation. Offer gratitude, converse, ask. After 1 minute, you may journal your observations.
6. **Awareness:** This practice need not be done in seated silence. Bring awareness to an everyday action such as walking or washing dishes. Notice what each of your senses picks up, the depth and rhythm of your breath, the passing thoughts. Do not be involved with it or judge it, just be aware. After 1 minute, you may journal your observations.

Now that you have tried all six types of meditation, spend a minute or two each day practicing the one that comes most naturally to you. Note that your meditation type may change over time.

As we mentioned before, the eightfold path of yoga, the yogic path of psychology, is sometimes called the "royal path." By having an external ethical code of restraints and an internal ethical code of observances, we become more discerning in how we treat others and, more importantly, ourselves. The uplifting attitudes of yoga postures, soothing effects of breathing practices, and sense mastery techniques support us in staying calm and understanding our own minds more deeply. This gives us the ability and commitment to remain aware throughout the day. By upholding focus in everyday life we begin to shape our thought patterns and brains to respond to life with less worry and feel dignified, empowered, and equipped to face life's challenges.

Chapter Summary

1. Meditation is a process to understand your own mind. Understanding removes stress and anxiety.
2. The ancient text *The Yoga Sutras of Patanjali* describes an eightfold path to peace. The eight limbs are:
    - Restraint of negative behavior (*Yama*)
    - Observance of positive behavior (*Niyama*)
    - Yoga postures (*Asana*)
    - Breathing and energy (*Pranayama*)
    - Sensory mastery (*Pratyahara*)
    - Concentration (*Dharana*)
    - Meditation (*Dhyana*)
    - Enlightenment (*Samadhi*)
3. The first limb is the restraint of harmful behaviors to self and others. The restraints are non-harm, truthfulness, non-stealing, moderation, and non-craving.

4. To avoid harming yourself with meditation, do not practice it if it causes more stress, spiraling thoughts, daydreaming, disassociation, or headaches. Do other mind-quieting activities instead.
5. The second limb of the eightfold path is observance of pure behaviors internally and externally. The observances are purity, contentment, discipline / effort, self-study, and surrender to a higher reality.
6. The third limb is the physical practices of yoga. The attitude we bring to yoga postures becomes stronger within us. Different poses inherently support different attitudes, such as courage, compassion, or surrender. Relaxation on an attitude is also beneficial.
7. The breath, the fourth limb, is linked to deeper states. Erratic, shallow breath is linked to chaotic thoughts and stress; steady breathing steadies the mind.
8. Our senses are bombarded each day. Withdrawing, or mastering, the senses is the fifth limb. Listening to a bird or relaxing music, gazing at a candle or nature, or warming up in a bath are all practices to draw the senses inward and quiet the mind.
9. There is a physiological reward in addition to the psychological dimension of anxiety: a dopamine response in the brain every time we are externally validated. This can lead to addictive behaviors. Because they are externally motivated, what you do to get rid of your anxiety can make it worse. This can include your postural and breathing habits.
10. Concentration, the sixth limb of the eightfold path, is about steadying the mind on a single subject. Any amount of effort here helps soothe stress, as the mind quiets and becomes clear.
11. Meditation, the seventh limb, is a state of pure concentration. There are six types of meditation: awareness or mindfulness of the present moment, plus five concentration styles: breath, visualization, mantra, prayer, and contemplation.

12. The eightfold path of yoga trains the mind to be still and limits its habit of creating stress through over-thinking. Strive to understand your mind, which helps clarify and balance situations.

This chapter taught you about important, fundamental concepts of the classical yoga path. Now you know a systematic way of understanding and gaining mastery over your lifestyle and state of mind. In the next chapter, we offer techniques to keep you from getting stuck in your head and intellectualizing the path. This way, you actually use the information to shift your inner and outer worlds in the direction of peace.

Chapter 6

The Yogic Path of the Intellect (Getting Out of Your Head)

We are in the information age. We know a great deal about many things. Because we know so much, most of us think too much and wind up stuck in our heads where all the information is. Inevitably, this over-thinking leads to stress and anxiety. This chapter teaches you the difference between knowing something and living from the truth of the information. The yogic path of the intellect recruits the power of information and harnesses it so that you are able to apply what you know and create a stress-free life.

Wisdom: From the Head to the Heart

If a stressed-out friend came to you looking for advice, you would not be lacking in suggestions! You are not at a loss for information on stress management. In a culture where stress is so prevalent, there is a wealth of data on dealing with it. If facts were all we required, none of us would be stressed anymore and anxiety would not be an international epidemic. What we actually need is beyond information.

One of the benefits of yoga is that it gives us a *direct experience* of eliminating stress and anxiety. The practice of yoga removes stress permanently, because it gives us a true experience of the higher self, the part of us that resides beyond stress. In other words, you know how to practice, then you do it, then you feel it, and then it is a part of you. The longest journey is from the head to the heart, from having information to integrating it into wisdom. We call this "realized knowledge."

When we are overcome with stress, we often seek solutions to our problems. This is a healthy impulse but can be taken too far when the quest for answers becomes a rehearsal of the problem. While some stressors require action, others need time to resolve. Some stress is inevitable, which entails acceptance. Thinking too much about our anxieties only makes them bigger. It is true that solutions often occur to us when we let go of the problem and give the mind space to relax. Yoga practices create space internally and externally. Turning to practice in times of stress shows wisdom—or realized knowledge—as we seek to unite with the unchanging, higher self rather than getting caught in a web of worries.

Think of a moment of happiness you experienced recently. Who was around you? What was happening? Why did it bring you joy? Usually, life's delights are small and simple, like watching birds at the feeder, finishing a project, sharing laughs with friends, or learning something new. Focusing on these joyful details helps inoculate us against stress. Notice, however, that we must be in a certain state of mind to perceive these details in the first place. The human brain assigns meaning so that we appreciate the beauty of life. If we are caught in the stress of survival mode, the reptilian brain focuses solely on its own selfish needs. On the other hand, establishing a daily routine that uplifts us helps set the tone of our entire lives.

The average person established in practice may go to bed early (practice starts the night before!) and wake up at the same time every day with a specific personal intention. The yoga mat is already laid out so it's easy to do a few poses or sit for breathing and meditation. A nourishing breakfast and connection with the family or spiritually uplifting reading may cap off the time at home. The drive to work may be in silence, or perhaps the commute is a carpool with friends, or a walk or bike ride through back trails. With the spiritual tone set so clearly, the higher self informs the events of the day. Challenges are faced without stress. The steady rhythm of each day supports a spiritual state of mind.

Exercise: Scheduling Care

As discussed above, when we bring spiritual attention to daily activities, we live with less stress and anxiety. This exercise helps you formulate a way to do this!

1. Consider the rhythm of your daily life and notice its effects on your overall sense of stress. What is your average daily schedule? Rough out a weekly or even monthly schedule to get a clear, honest picture of where your time is going and what your priorities are. Does your schedule reflect your commitment to yoga practice, self-care, or removing anxiety?
2. When does your self-care/higher self fit into your schedule? Where could you insert 10 minutes of yoga practice into an average day?
3. Is it possible to bring your higher self into jobs that are not exclusively for yourself? For example, housework is making a beautiful home and training a new employee is an opportunity for kindness and connection. How can your higher self be present no matter what you are doing? In 30 seconds, write down as many ways as you can think of.

Exercise: Present Times

This exercise helps you become more present in everyday life. Take a few moments now to contemplate the stressful moments in your schedule and how you might soothe them through insight.

1. Building off the schedule from the previous exercise, become aware of the rise and fall of your stress levels through an average day. You may gain more insights if you repeat this enquiry for one week.
2. When are you most stressed? What time of day are you most vulnerable to feeling anxious? This is your peak stress time each day.

3. What insights arose regarding your life or personality, simply by noticing your stress level through the day? Similarly, what did you learn about yourself from observing these daily patterns? Repeat this exercise over a few days for more insights.

Exercise: Evaluating and Responding

This sequence of exercises is helping you figure out how to alleviate stress in a conscious way. Now is the time to call on your intellect to understand your deeper triggers and unwind the daily peaks of stress and anxiety.

1. Reflecting on the pattern of your peak stress time, brainstorm some reasons why it might be occurring when it is. Remember to look at the big picture of your daily and weekly schedule to understand all the lifestyle factors at play.
2. What was happening 10 minutes prior to the peak stress time? When was the last time you ate? How tired were you? Who else was present? How about 30 minutes, 60 minutes, even 2 hours before the peak stress time?
3. Knowing the peak stress time is approaching, you may begin to observe your breathing and thought patterns before the stress actually peaks. Begin to apply practices to intervene so that the stress diminishes rather than climaxes.

Relying on our practice marks the difference between knowing what to do, actually doing it, and being established in it. The yogic path of the intellect is about more than knowing; it is about experiencing. You can think of it like describing what a peach tastes like to someone who has never eaten one. There are no adjectives to capture its specific quality of sweetness, its soft outer fuzz, or the silky, wet insides when it's perfectly ripe. Imagine continuing to explain the difference in flavors between fresh and canned peaches, yellow and white, Georgia and Ontario. Words cannot express these subtle delights. You might wonder,

Why are we on a tangent about peaches? The simple reason is to say, *Just eat a peach!* There is little point in describing what cannot be known, of *thinking* about what must be *experienced*. Meditation, lifestyle practices, and stress-free living are like that, as well. Realized knowledge means doing it—having a direct experience of it—and then it becomes a part of you.

The Reason for Stress

Our beliefs are the foundation upon which all of our decisions are made. In some regard, beliefs are the lenses through which we view reality; paradoxically, they prevent us from seeing reality for what it is. Beliefs are very much *our* truths, but not *the* Truth. Beliefs—arising from our society, family, education, religion, experience—feed our desires and habits. If we deeply hold a version of reality that is a certain way, we will act in accordance with it; it is stressful not to act on the belief because of our limited perception. Over time, repeating these actions based on the same preconceived ideas, we become established in habits, whether or not they truly serve the higher self. The habits arose to serve our desires and belief systems, based on our level of understanding.

The trouble that arises is, except in very rare circumstances, our beliefs do not explain reality correctly. Although there may be facets of truth within our perceptions, they tend to be too biased to accurately reflect reality. When the beliefs incorrectly explain any part of reality, we feel a dissonance of disconnection from the higher self, who lives in pure truth. Doubt arises out of that disconnection from truth. For most of us, our treasured beliefs operate below conscious radar. In fact, many self-serving desires—and even some selfless ones—do a good job of keeping themselves hidden.

Once we realize a belief, we are able to edit it. Beliefs are continually changing, either through conscious effort or through not-conscious processes of integrating learning. The following are some common belief statements. How truly do you feel that they describe reality? The first statement is a commonly expressed perspective. The second version offers a more reality-based perspective.

Common Belief	Reality-Based Perspective
I am not good enough.	I give my best effort.
I should be perfect.	I discover my talents by trial and error.
I am unlovable.	I accept myself for who I am now.
I need to look this way for others to like me.	I appreciate myself from the inside out.

We will always have beliefs. Without them we may become aloof, indecisive, or unproductive; without beliefs we have no foundation. How can we use them to create a life of well-being rather than stress? We are moving in the direction of realized knowledge, where our beliefs are based on direct experience and higher perspective, not lowly programming, hopes, expectations, or fears. The yogic path of the intellect teaches that it is important to explore and refine our beliefs and understanding.

Exercise: Analyzing Expectations

This exercise can help get you out of stressful habits by exploring and understanding your hidden beliefs. The more you work with your beliefs, the more you know how well you are able to shake free of them.

1. Off the cuff, write out what you expect from yourself and life. Do not censor yourself, no matter how unreasonable your list comes out. Take only 30 seconds to create this unfiltered list, after which time you may begin to analyze and interfere with pure experience.
2. Review this list of expectations. Are there any surprises? Can you see how some of your unhealthy habits arise directly from these beliefs? What happens to your stress levels when you see these expectations?
3. Create another list, based on the first, which purifies your beliefs as demonstrated in the chart above. For example, "I

am trapped by this situation" becomes "I am the creator of my internal experience," and "I don't try because I might fail. What a waste of my effort," becomes "If I do my best, I can't fail because the pure effort is worthy."

Spiritual Reading

Do you take time to read? If so, what do you read? Is it novels, scientific journals, self-help books, magazines, spiritual works, newspapers, Internet articles, children's books? Reading can help quiet the mind; however, the content of some books can actually create more anxiety. In fact, some reading material may be more disturbing than television, which is very disruptive to peace of mind. While reading is definitely a break from the stresses of reality and harshness of blue screens, not all books are created equal. Nonfiction, philosophical, and spiritual texts tend to create the fewest internal disruptions as they appeal to the higher self and our sense of truth. Such texts can offer meaningful perspectives, cause for reflection, and even focal points for meditation. Within the observances of yoga, as discussed previously, we are guided to read spiritual works as an aspect of internal purity. Which specific books uplift and soothe you? The yogic path of the intellect asks us to study and gather pure, deeply true information so that we can apply it to the action of our everyday lives.

Exercise: Let Others Uplift You

Books can be an excellent anti-anxiety tool. Even thousands of years ago the sages recommended study as a path to ease and wisdom. Just a little bit of reading from a pure source each day can activate the imagination and set thoughts in the direction of well-being.

1. Select a book that makes you feel reassured and happy. This can be scripture, self-help, poetry, fiction, or even stories from childhood. The important thing is that you are reading something that gives you a clear perspective on the goodness of life and your own value and purpose.

2. Read a short passage from the book every day. Let the words lull you to sleep. As you go through your day, be aware of how you can apply the message of your reading to everyday life. Look for ways to bring a deeper meaning into your everyday activities—you will find them!

When You've Heard It Before

Shelly, a dedicated yoga student, was sure to attend at least one workshop every season as a way of deepening practice. In these workshops Shelly could often be heard expressing, "I've done that exercise before, so there wasn't much for me to learn" or "I heard that before so I already knew it." Shelly believed that if something was not new information, it didn't contribute to personal growth. This limiting belief robbed Shelly of years of self-study and development. Unfortunately, painful and unhealthy habits continued in Shelly's life for years. It wasn't until Shelly began comparing everyday actions to the repeated information that true transformation occurred. Now, Shelly is grateful for the gift of repetition and measures personal progress against familiar practices and hearing the same ideas and information again.

There are only a few simple truths in life. These truths are expressed across religions and over long periods of time. Those of us on a personal growth path are not seeking data; we are seeking a direct experience of what those truths are suggesting. In other words, we are not looking for information; we are on a quest for realized knowledge.

Why read the same texts over and over? Many of the core texts of yoga remind us that realized knowledge—be it happiness, enlightenment, freedom from stress, or whatever you specifically seek—arises from constant practice over a long period of time. By revisiting the same inspiring texts, attending classes and trainings, sharing with like-minded friends, we learn to discern more of a deeper truth every time. We shift from thinking about the higher self to living in alignment with its truth. This is truly transformational!

If you have been battling stress or anxiety for a long time, you have likely heard similar recommendations again and again. Breathe deeply, accept yourself, take time every day for self-care, eat well, rest... There are only a few, simple truths in life. These fundamental truths are constant; however, *we* are constantly changing. Even when we hear the same recommendation for the hundredth time, we are one hundred times different. This is the gift of repetition. Do not shirk repeated information just because you have heard it before. Ask yourself: What am I doing with this information? How have I applied it to my everyday life? How have my habits changed since I first heard the information? There is a vast difference between knowing something intellectually and demonstrating understanding by actually living in alignment with what we know.

The hallmark of one with realized knowledge is that they have shifted from having the information to using it. They have gone from knowing to doing. Wisdom is reflected in their routines and lifestyle choices, in all the areas where they possess this realized knowledge. Daily habits offer us all stability, consistency, and the comfort of a framework holding the day together. Conversely, internal chatter sets tone of each moment, no matter what the events of the day. In a state of realized knowledge, we are able to acknowledge that stressful internal chatter without becoming involved with it. The voice of wisdom within us is able to discern between the worried, judgmental lower self and the pure, connected higher self, and it is the latter that we trust.

Exercise: Belief Habits

There is great power in this next exercise, which investigates your mental habits and story to root out where you are not living according to what you know. In other words, you can discover the gap in your realized knowledge. From there, we build a bridge so that you are empowered to live in accordance with the person you want to be and what you know to be true.

1. Honestly list your daily habits that contribute to feeling stress or anxiety. Going to bed too late, participating in addictions, berating ourselves, and isolating from friends are some common examples of stress-creating behaviors. It is okay to have these weaknesses; the next step is to be aware of them.

2. What is the belief system that pervades these habits or choices? Record the "story" you tell yourself about why you make these choices. Remain truthful and do not judge yourself. The point of this is to understand the roots of unhealthy actions. Some enabling beliefs include:
   - "I've had a rough day."
   - "No one else thinks this behavior is a problem."
   - "I'm healthy in other areas of my life."
3. Write an affirmation that addresses the enabling belief systems. Allow these affirmations to support you in making conscious, balanced everyday choices. Sometimes you will choose the stress-producing behavior; however, in time these affirmations will counter the beliefs behind the choices. By addressing the roots of the unhealthy habits, the behavior itself will change. Affirmations relating to above statements may be:
   - "I care for myself in loving ways (especially after a rough day)."
   - "I listen to myself and choose behaviors that keep me well."
   - "I balance my life with health."
4. Select one habit from the list you made in Step 1 that contributes to your stress or anxiety. List some small, positive steps that you can take to shift the habit. In this way, you strengthen your mental health and move in the direction of realized knowledge.

Exercise: Variety in Yoga Postures

Sometimes one of the best things we can do to engage the intellect for change is perform something familiar in a completely different way. This exercise takes the posture sequence from Chapter 1 and has you approach the yoga poses differently. Notice how varying the approach opens your mind to new possibilities of experience.

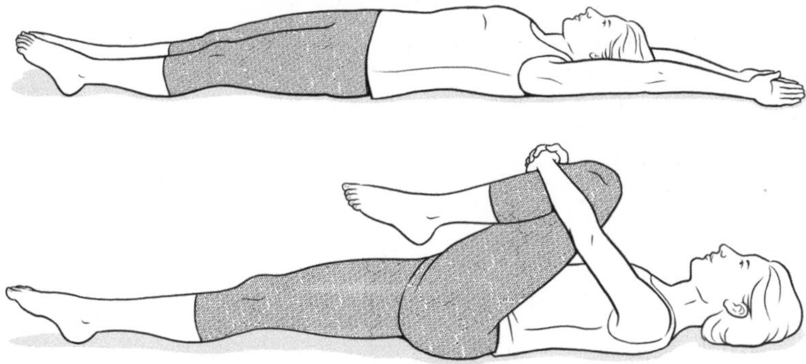

Figure 6.1a and 6.1b
1. *Yastikasana/Pavana Muktasana* (**Stick Pose/Wind-Releasing Pose**)

Exhale to raise both arms overhead, placing the back of your hands on the floor overhead. Reach out from the waist and middle back in either direction to make your body as long as possible while keeping your shoulders relaxed (*Yastikasana*). Inhale, pull your toes toward the sky, and draw your right knee toward your chest, holding gently with both hands either at the shin or behind the knee (preferably the opposite to your usual habit) (*Pavana Muktasana*). Repeat the exhale, reaching your body long and open into *Yastikasana.* Inhale the other (left) knee to the chest, holding with both hands while your heels press outward and toes reach up. Think of initiating the movement from your hands and on the next repetition from your feet. This won't look any different, but it does engage your brain differently.

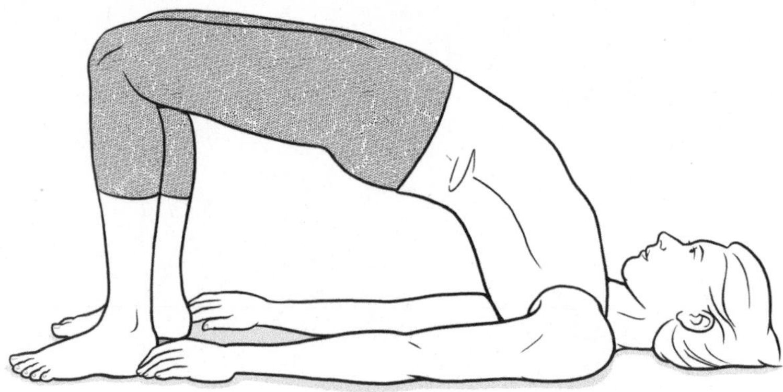

Figure 6.2
2. *Setu Bandhasana* (**Bridge Pose**)

Rest on your back and bend your knees, bringing them hip-width apart with your feet planted close to your buttocks. Ensure feet and knees remain in line with the hips through the entire pose rather than collapsing them in or out. *Exhale* and lift, rather than roll, the pelvis upward from the mat. Imagine that you are being pushed upward from behind, rather than pulled upward from the front (or vice versa if that is already your habit). Hold for a comfortable time, breathing regularly and grounding into your legs and feet before lowering on an *inhale* as if the push from behind were getting softer and the pull from gravity getting stronger.

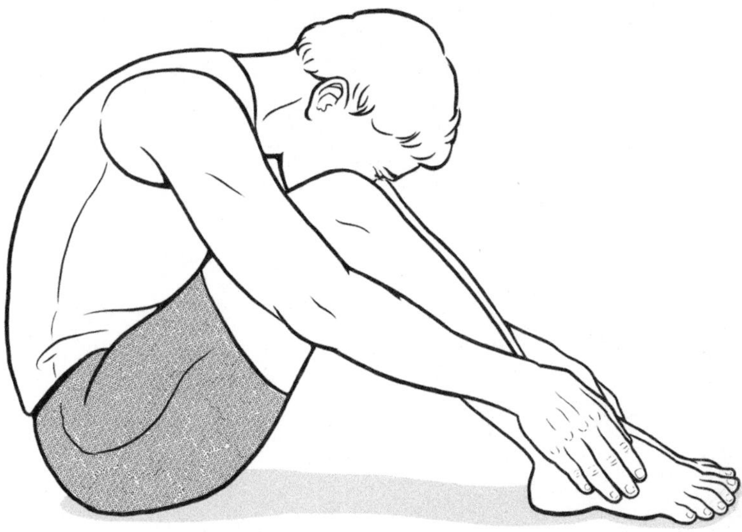

Figure 6.3
3. Restorative Forward Bend

Come to a seated position. Soles of the feet on the floor, similar to the posture above, *inhale* and rest the front of your body on the front of your thighs, resting your forehead on your knees. You may need to fold your arms on your knees to create a pillow for your head; otherwise, rest them alongside the legs. Become aware of the breath moving along the back of your body. After a few breaths imagine it moving along the front of your body. Roll up gently, looking down all the while.

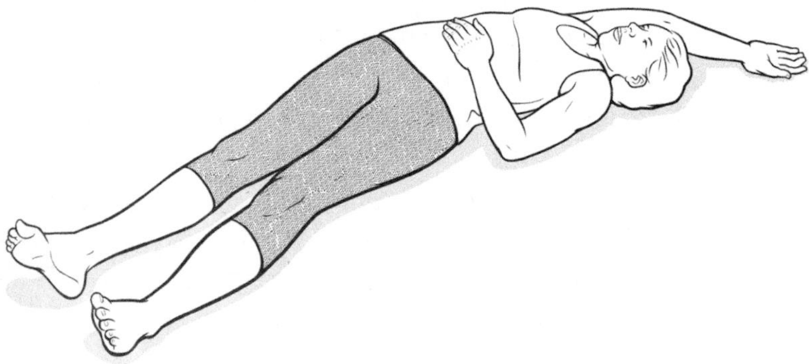

Figure 6.4
4. *Supta Ardha Chandrasana* (**Supine Half-Moon Pose**)

Straighten your legs out along the floor and walk your feet to right side, raising *your right arm overhead*, the back of your hand resting on the floor (bend the elbow if necessary). Notice your breath and sensation in the *left* (compressed) side of the body. Repeat on the other side.

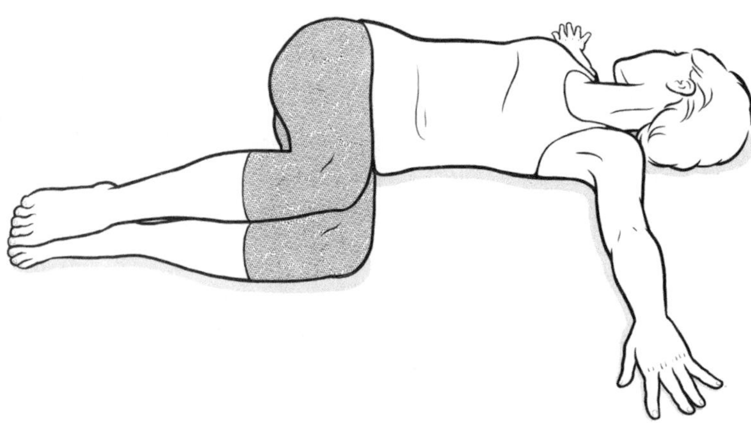

Figure 6.5
5. *Supta Matsyendrasana* (**Reclined Half Twist**)

Extend your arms to the sides in a "T" position at shoulder height and bring your knees into the chest, facing the palms *upward* (or, if that is your usual habit, face them to the floor). To protect your back, keep your feet on the floor at all times; otherwise, your knees can go right into your chest. *Inhale* the legs to one side and ensure that your feet are supported by the earth. If you are free from neck issues, turn your face lightly in the opposite direction of the knees. You may straighten your legs along the floor for variety, aiming to have them at a right angle to the torso. *Exhale* to come out of the pose. Repeat on the other side.

Even small adjustments in how we approach our postures—or anything in life!—can shift our awareness and open us to new, creative understanding. When we get stuck in our heads, it can be very helpful to slightly alter our way of doing things in order to effect and integrate change in our lives. The following exercise teaches you how to discern what areas may be ready to change.

Exercise: Decoding the Body Scan

There was a time in your life before stress and anxiety. There were times when you have felt worry or even fear and not been consumed or debilitated by it. You are learning tools and practicing skills to transcend stress and anxiety. Simple practices in everyday life are key to shifting perspectives, coming home to the body, and aligning with the higher self. The following exercise helps attune you to underlying perspectives being expressed through the body and gives you a path of self-enquiry so that you can receive the messages and improve your life.

1. Perform a body scan relaxation (from Chapter 4) by slowly scanning your body from the crown of your head to the soles of your feet, suggesting sequentially that all areas relax. This scanning can best be described as bringing full awareness to whatever part of the body you are paying attention to.
2. Notice which areas of the body are reluctant to let go of tension. Sometimes our bodies give us clues about what is going on beyond conscious awareness. The following enquiry can offer insight into what beliefs, likes, dislikes, desires, and expectations may be blocked from your intellectual awareness.

3. Reflect on the following enquiry: What was the quality of tension in the resistant places you found in the body? How is the tension there interacting with the rest of your body? If the tension could speak, what would it say? If it was there to give you a message, what message would it want you to receive? If it had a need, what need might it be trying to express? If this resistant tension were a small child who required care, in what ways could you lovingly respond? You will get more out of this exercise if you journal your responses.

Exercise: "When I die…"

You are going to die. Don't worry—so is everyone else! Accepting this fact actually helps lessen anxiety. None of us wants to look back on life from its end and realize we spent most of our time focusing on what did not matter. When we truly embrace the idea that death is a part of living, we are able to make decisions in the context of this wisdom. The following exercise helps give perspective.

1. Whenever you feel stress arising, remember that you will be dead in a few decades and that report, chore, relationship, or transgression will no longer matter. All you have to do is give the best of your efforts and character to every day, knowing it may be the last. Be careful: this is not a dark, ominous thought but rather a pure, freeing awareness of truth!
2. How might your awareness of death change your life? When we remember that we will soon be gone, there is more tenderness and attention in life. We no longer wait to tell people we love them. We resolve quarrels quickly. We don't put off our dreams. Although initially contemplating our own death feels uncomfortable, scary, even morbid, death is simply a fact of life. Acceptance of this fact helps us live more fully.
3. What was the biggest stress you encountered today? Answer the same question for this week, this month, this year, and

the past five years. Review the list and beside each stress write "Yes" or "No" to the question, "Will this matter at the end of my life?" What we know from speaking to many elders is that for most of us what will matter in the end is how we nurtured the soul: how closely we aligned with our purpose, the quality of our work and relationships, our contributions to society. Relax and connect to the higher self, trusting this aspect of you to offer guidance around what is truly important.

4. The next time you feel stressed or upset, ask yourself, will this matter in the end?

Exercise: Your Higher Self

1. Practice the body scan relaxation (taught in Chapter 4 and described briefly above) to soothe your mind and enhance inner awareness.
2. As you relax, allow your mind to drift to a time in childhood—a moment when you felt completely whole, peaceful, and engaged ... a time when you felt completely safe. You may be alone in this moment or with others; that is not important. What is important is that deep feeling of connection, awareness, and wonder. It may be sitting in a tree, watching the ripples of a lake, or laughing with friends. It may be resting in a loving hug or hearing a beautiful melody; whatever connects you to a deep feeling is correct.
3. Write about this time in as much detail as you can, calling on all of your senses and feelings to recreate the experience and document it. (Alternatively you may draw or paint it with as much feeling as possible.)
4. Read over this paragraph a few times, slowly, to deepen your remembrance of this sacred moment in your life. In this moment, through this memory, you are connected to your higher self. Whatever you were doing made you happy, which is to say close to your natural state of peacefulness, love, and ease. At that time in memory, your stressors were far away

from you and you felt an awareness of something greater than the everyday. Perhaps, even now, as you read your writing, your everyday stressors seem a little further away.

5. You may practice this exercise repeatedly, excavating many powerful moments from the course of your life.

Stress and Anxiety Are Your Best Friends

The discomfort of stress is a reminder that we have forgotten the higher self. Stress and anxiety, therefore, serve as reminders of the higher self! Feeling out of sorts can be a trigger to rebalance ourselves. When we allow the anxiety and stress to remind us to call upon the higher self, then that stress becomes a good friend and great tool on the path of enlightenment! Wise people still encounter stress, they simply apply realized knowledge to the situation, reconnect, and proceed with balance and calm.

By recruiting the power of your intellect, you can transcend stress. The yogic path of the intellect reminds us that shifting from *having* information to *using* it will change your life. Living in accordance with your deep, true beliefs and communing with the higher self is uplifting and empowering. Ultimately, the power of realized knowledge supports us in changing our habits, understanding why we really do what we do, and offers the perspective needed to let go of stress and anxiety.

Chapter Summary

1. Realized knowledge arises from the experience of doing something and cannot be taught in any other way.
2. Thinking too much about problems causes problems.
3. Daily rhythm helps us restrain unhealthy impulses, regulate desires, accept internal authority, and achieve personal mastery.
4. Understanding daily rhythms of stress empowers us to intervene with practices such as deep breathing, discerning thought patterns, and yoga postures before the stress actually peaks.
5. Life's delights are small, simple, and free.

6. Beliefs, even ones we are not aware of, color our perception of life and decisions. Once we are aware of our underlying beliefs, we can shape them based on higher perspectives.
7. Spiritual reading uplifts us and teaches us about ourselves.
8. There are a few simple truths in life. They don't change. We do. Move beyond information to the realm of understanding and acting appropriately.
9. Wisdom reveals itself through simple, healthy, daily routines. Discover your own rhythms of ease and peace of mind.
10. Anxiety-driven routines stem from beliefs. Applying wisdom to enabling statements makes it harder for us to lie to ourselves, then we change the belief through affirmation and behavior.
11. You have faced stress in the past without anxiety; you can do so again. Listen to what your body is trying to tell you about your holistic needs.
12. Reflecting on times when you felt aligned with your higher self draws it closer to the surface. Study your own peak experiences and meaningful moments, applying the wisdom and feeling of those times to everyday life.
13. Accept stress and anxiety as reminders of the higher self. When they arise, rather than dwell on the worry, use it as a cue to reconnect.

The next chapter moves us out of the mind and into the body. While the intellect is a valid and beneficial path out of stress and anxiety, the body offers us concrete tools to minimize those symptoms as well.

Chapter 7

The Yogic Path of Health

This chapter looks at health via two main perspectives: the energy of the whole person—with a special focus on breath—and nutrition for the whole person. Classical yoga's comprehensive lifestyle approach revitalizes ancient methods to include the physical, energetic, mental, intellectual, and spiritual health. This is the yogic path of health. In this chapter we are going to apply the five layers of a person (*koshas*) to personal health and minimizing stress and anxiety. The five layers of a person, which we discussed in the previous chapter, moving from obvious to subtle, are body, life energy / breath, mind / feeling, intellect, and spirit / higher self. We will explore how we can use the ancient healing techniques on each of your layers to bring balance by considering healthy nutrition for the whole person.

Eat to nourish your body, energy, mind, intellect, and spirit. When Comprehensive Yoga Therapists teach nutrition, the paradigm includes more than just the physical food we eat. Nutrition for the whole person considers everything we are taking in. It is important to realize that each layer of our beings requires nutrition. In other words, we feed ourselves on all levels. We are continually taking in from the world around us; once we are aware of this, we may be more discerning about our interactions with the world around us. The boundaries between the physical body, breath, mind, intellect, and spiritual layers are permeable. The body and mind are balanced by deep breathing. Uplifting emotions give spiritual joy. Stimulating learning causes the mind to develop and guide life in creative directions. Spiritual practices lend emotional and intellectual inspiration and direction. Thus, the appropriate reason for eating is to experience the highest states of consciousness. Throughout the day, we feed ourselves on many levels. Similarly, the food that we eat has a relationship with all layers of our being. Our physical, energetic, mental, intellectual, and spiritual states all influence our food choices, and the food we ingest impacts our well-being. This chapter discusses the importance of healthy life energy by focusing on the importance of breath and nutrition for the whole person.

Health Explained

Before modern medicine came along we had to rely solely on herbs, food, rest, water, community, and ancient healing practices to maintain health. There was very little chronic stress in the world at that time, but life expectancy was short—modern medicine has definitely made a difference! We have better access to food and clean water, and the progress of modern medicine has helped us with various disease conditions. But ironically, the modern world has brought with it a long life filled with stress and anxiety. It is almost comical that the decrease in ancient practices that didn't allow for a long life came from a time when the quality of life was high and stress was low. Before the advent of the home computer, children never said they were stressed. Children in the 1970s or 1980s, before the Internet, wouldn't have known the word "stress," yet in today's world, most children will say they are stressed for one reason or another. Unlike our modern medicine, ancient healing methods are based on creating balance. We can use some of these ancient methods to rid ourselves of stress so we can benefit from modern medicine and live a long life stress-free. Let's do both!

Anxious people often suffer from similar health conditions. Nervous system disorders, heart conditions, chronic pain, digestive diseases, autoimmune conditions, sleep disorders, mental health concerns, and many other issues are associated with or worsened by anxiety and stress. While yoga's goal is not only physical, it does confer distinct, powerful benefits to the body. The sense of ease, peace, and well-being from practicing yoga postures results from a harmonization, revitalization, and balancing of all the systems of the body, most notably the nervous system, the musculoskeletal system, the hormonal system, and the healthy circulation of lymph, blood, oxygen, and life energy. Yoga postures and practices can limit the deleterious effects of stress on health.

Traditional yoga practices are a path to steadiness of mind. By connecting with ultimate concepts and experiencing profound peace, contentment, and acceptance, we learn to hold a connection to the higher self through everyday trials. This higher perspective can be likened to a person standing at an overlook, viewing a busy scene from a distance. There is an awareness of the busyness, its causes and effects, but the viewer is not involved. As we gain a broader perspective, our mental and psychological habits become clear. Through this clarity we can let go of stress and connect to what is more important. This shift in mental and spiritual state is often reported as the most healing aspect of yoga therapy. In this book we discuss the benefits separately; however, realize that we achieve freedom from stress through a holistic, balanced approach to yoga. The Yogic Path of Health reminds us that we must manage our stress levels, get sufficient rest, and consistently eat nutritious whole foods. These practices help balance our vital life energy.

Chakras or Life Energy Centers

We each have a life energy field that surrounds us; in scientific terms this is recognized as a measurable electromagnetic field, like the earth's north and south poles. Our neural activity is similarly electromagnetic. Yoga poses strengthen the vertebral column and the trunk of the body, improving the function of the central energetic channel and nervous system communication. As we develop body awareness, we may begin to notice the subtle flow of energy during a yoga pose in the form of warmth, tingling, or mental imagery. Locked joints and muscular tension trap anxious energy in the body and limit the circulation of blood, lymph, and life energy. Once we recognize the sense of energy flow, we can begin to consciously direct it, helping us to achieve greater health.

While modern medicine has made great strides in knowledge about the physical systems of the body, ancient medicine has a much more sophisticated understanding of the body's energetic system. Historically, the former studied cadavers while the latter researched health through living organisms. The life energy system described in yoga is comprised of seven major energy centers or wheels (*chakras*), the meridians it flows through (*nadis*), and the life energy itself (*prana*). Chakras, nadis, and prana can relate to the anatomical concepts of nerve plexi, nerves, and nerve impulses.

The concept of life energy centers appeared in modern literature in the fourteenth century. These life energy centers address the human being in terms of body, mind, and spirit. The heart chakra, for example, corresponds to the anatomical heart, the thalamus gland, feelings of love, the color green, the element of air, and spiritual devotion. These life energy centers have unique physical associations where subtle life energy is absorbed and distributed to the cells, organs, and tissues. It is generally understood that there are seven major energy centers, which have some association with the nerve plexus and endocrine glands, but more specifically with the Chinese system of acupuncture meridians.

Body posture can be one of the more obvious links to these centers. An example is the solar plexus center, located at the base of the ribcage. When someone is lacking confidence, the body slumps as if punched in the stomach. The middle back curves forward, rounding the shoulders and neck forward and down. From a bio-energetic standpoint, this particular body posture blocks the flow of energy through the solar plexus, which limits connection to a sense of confidence and purpose. Consider the effect this could have on stress levels! A slumped posture lowers energy, while an upright posture uplifts the mind, strengthens the core (both physically and metaphorically) and facilitates deep breathing. By lifting out of the abdomen and middle back, the solar plexus automatically opens, improving the flow of energy and imbuing an innate confidence.

Exercise: Chakra Focus Through Yoga

When practicing yoga postures, it's easy to overemphasize the physical aspects of the practice. Life energy centers (*chakras*) offer us a wonderful opportunity to concentrate on the spiritual and emotional aspects of yoga postures, and, as such, are an important part of a balanced yoga practice. As we develop subtle awareness in the postures, we practice on an entirely different level—one far more enriching and vitalizing. As you discover how to sense your life energy and begin balancing it, you will realize significant benefits in your daily life.

1. Bring this chakra awareness into your yoga pose practice by selecting the location of one chakra (base of spine, low belly/sacrum, solar plexus, heart, throat, third eye, or top of head) and witness it throughout the practice of the postures below. Note: You can bring this chakra focus to any yoga practice you do.
2. Notice the subtle sensations that occur. See how focus on that specific area influences your approach to postures, as well as your breath, emotions, and thoughts.
3. The following is a sample practice you can use, holding focus on any one of the seven major energy centers. Remember that you can use a life energy focus during any yoga pose practice; the following is just one of infinite practice possibilities.
    - Begin by warming up the body with gentle movements and joint rotations, or by going for a walk.

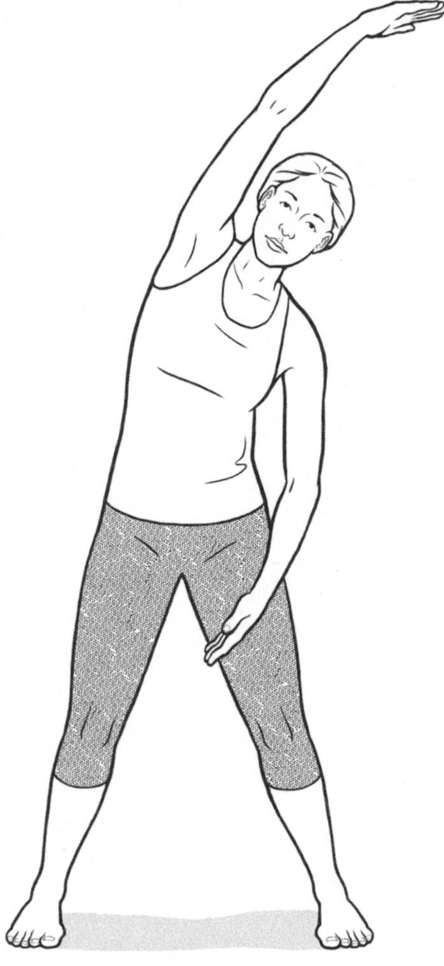

Figure 7.1
Standing Side Bend

Place feet wider than hip-width and protect your back by keeping your hips square, not pushed out to either side. On an exhale, bend into the soft part of your waist, shortening the distance between the side of your lowest rib and your hip. The top arm may be raised to increase stretch. Inhale back to center and repeat on the other side.

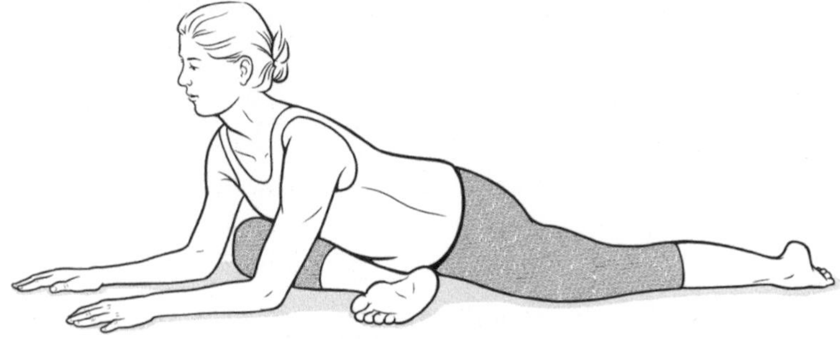

Figure 7.2
Eka Pada Kapotasana (**Pigeon Pose**)

From all fours (hands and knees), slide your right knee forward and place it between your hands, then set your right hip and thigh down while tucking your foot toward the groin. Straighten your left leg out directly behind you. The left knee may be more comfortable rotated open to the left side rather than down to the floor. Lift your chest, extend your spine, and arch to a slight backbend. Hold the core strong to protect your back. If your back is comfortable, your right arm may reach out in front at shoulder height or lift up alongside your ear. Repeat on the other side.

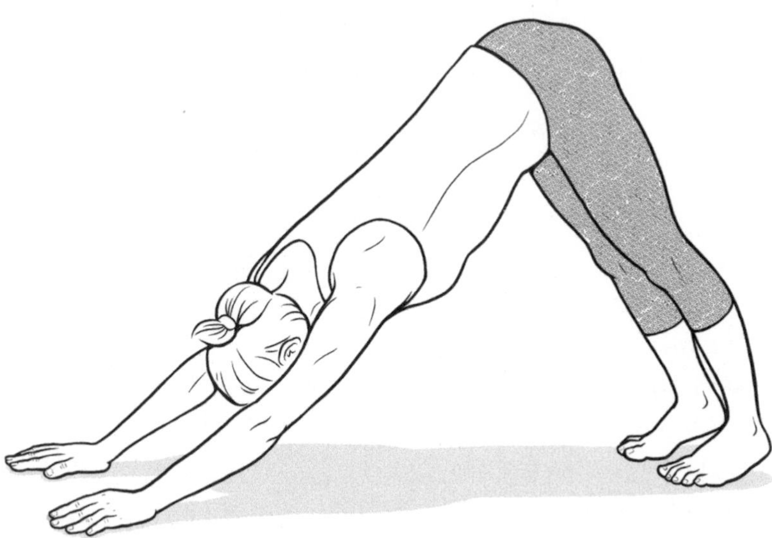

Figure 7.3
Adho Mukha Svanasana (**Downward-Facing Dog Pose**)

It is an option to apply this pose as a transition between Pigeon Pose on the left and right sides of your body. If appropriate for you, bring your hands on either side of the bent leg in Pigeon and turn your toes under behind you. Then press into the back foot and hands, lifting the hips up as your chest presses forward and down. The bent, front leg straightens out behind so the body is in the shape of a symmetrical triangle, with the hips as the highest point. Spread your fingers, pressing into your fingertips, and lengthen your heels toward the floor. Come into Pigeon on the other side by bringing the opposite knee between the hands and gently lowering the hips to the floor.

Alternatively, practice Downward-Facing Dog after you have completed Pigeon on both sides by coming to your hands and knees, then pressing into hands and feet, straighten the knees and lift the hips up and back, aiming them at the place where the wall meets the ceiling behind you, all the while lengthening your heels.

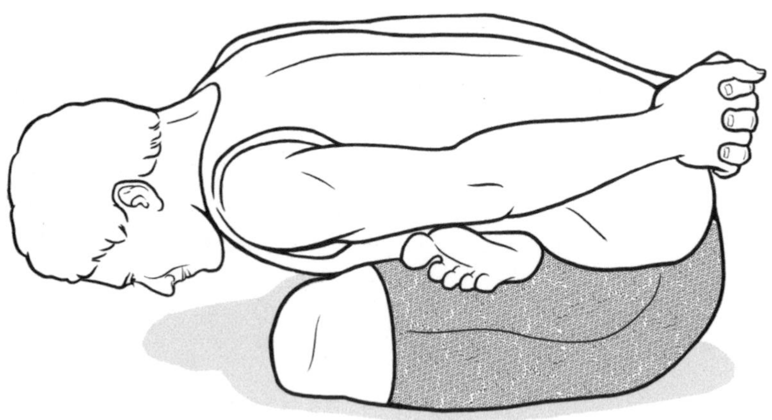

Figure 7.4
Yoga Mudra **(Symbol of Yoga)**

From a comfortable seated position such as cross-legged, clasp your hands behind your body, keeping your arms relaxed. Twist left and roll the torso forward as far as your body will comfortably allow, as if to bring forehead to knee. Your back may be rounded. Inhale to sit tall then repeat with a twist to the right. You may perform the posture one more time directly to the center. Allow body and breath to relax as deeply as possible.

Mind/Body Health Through the Breath

We just discussed the life energy effects on your body. You may have noticed that tuning in on this level has an effect on the state of your mind/feelings. This section tunes you in to how your energetic nutrition, via the breath, affects your mental state. An interesting experiment can be to observe how you breathe at different times during the day. Connect the way your breathing patterns influence your state of mind and vice versa. Notice the subtle physical sensations when you are anxious, how your body seems to spin or is light or erratic. After doing a breathing practice, notice a sense of being settled and balanced in body, life energy/breath, and mind/feelings. It is beneficial to "feed" ourselves a healthy breath.

The amount of nutrition derived from breathing is very important as most of us would die in a matter of minutes without breath. However, through conscious direction of the breath, we can connect the five layers of our being, from the physical through the spiritual. Conscious breath control can transform you at every level, supporting mental balance and freedom from stress. In yoga there is a saying that we are given a certain number of breaths in life and in order to live to an old age we have to be sure to make each breath as long as possible!

Exercise: Breath Self-Analysis

Anxiety clearly shows itself in the way we breathe. Rapid, shallow, or erratic breathing instantly triggers a stress response through the entire body. By understanding our breathing habits, we can begin to intervene on our own behalf and keep the nervous system balanced, thereby holding anxiety at bay. Even if you are a longtime yoga student and understand your breathing patterns, act as if you were a beginner observing breathing for the first time and enjoy the opportunity to learn about the relationship between your psyche and breathing habits from this exercise.

1. Sit or stand in a habitual "bad posture" of yours. You may imagine your form at the computer or on the couch at the end of a long day. Even though you know this posture is unhealthy, hold it as you observe:
2. What parts of your lungs (diaphragm, ribs, upper chest) move while you are in this position and which are restricted? How many seconds is each inhale and each exhale? What about the pauses between these breath phases? What is the quality of the breathing? Is it choppy? Does it move in stages like an elevator? Or start fast, then slow, or vice versa?
3. What is happening through the rest of your body as you hold this position and breathe this way? How is your pelvis, back, neck, shoulders? How about your limbs, hands, and feet? What is your face expressing? Don't judge or change it; just observe. To assist in understanding, you may use your arms and hands to exaggerate the feeling associated with this breathing pattern.
4. What emotions arise in relation to this breath? What is the speed, quality, and content of your thoughts? How do your thoughts change as you continue slouching and witnessing breath?
5. Now settle into a tall, comfortable posture that embodies dignity. Witness the breath and ask yourself the above questions again.

Although it requires some muscular engagement to hold ourselves tall, we tend to be more emotionally and mentally relaxed. Conversely, many of us think we are relaxing when we slouch. This exercise shows that even when we think we are doing something to relax, we are actually creating an internal climate of stress by constricting the breath. Try this in life: the next time you feel tired or stressed, draw yourself up to your full height, deepen your breath, and watch the anxiety dissipate!

Exercise: Life Energy and Breath

In yoga philosophy, it is believed that breath is the vehicle for life energy. All cultural traditions of the world describe the breath in a spiritual manner as breath gives life. Life energy can perhaps best be understood as a combination of vitality and breath. Our life energy is affected by our choices and experiences, whether physical, emotional, or spiritual in nature. You can witness this in yourself via the following brief exercise.

1. Without changing anything, notice your breathing and vitality right now. What is the breath's depth and rhythm? Is it smooth or choppy? Are there pauses in the breath? Is it comfortable? Do you feel relaxed, energized, and clear, or tense, drained, and foggy?
2. Think of a situation that has been causing you stress lately. Notice what happens to your sense of vitality and your breathing pattern by asking similar questions to those in Step 1.
3. Think of an uplifting, comforting, or pleasant experience. Repeat similar enquiries to those in Step 1. How were your breathing and sense of vitality different when you were thinking of a stressor versus this happy thought? By directing your mind, you have power over the subtle aspects of your energy and health!

Breathing exercises can also help us connect with the healing qualities of our life energy. As we know, the solar plexus represents personal purpose, motivation, and confidence. By connecting the breath with feelings of service and effort, we can discover a new level of awareness in yoga postures. An example of linking breath and energetic intention in Warrior Pose is to view inhalation as a way of fortifying strength and courage, and exhalation as a way of giving service and good works to others. By practicing in this way, you'll likely feel a greater sense of connection to others and to yourself. Be creative in your breathing and posture visualizations—they truly enhance well-being.

Our life energy processes and "remembers" emotional events. This appears to be an important contributing factor, along with heredity, diet, exposure to environmental toxins, bacteria, and viruses, to why some people get ill and others do not. Life energy may be the weakest link in the chain, as it is typically the first to break under emotional and spiritual stress.

Exercise: Clarifying the Energy of Stress

According to the yogic path of health, our stressful thoughts, feelings, and physiological reactions are all connected and expressed through our life energy. Because life energy is subtle, many of us cannot relate to it directly, and instead must call in the body or mind to help the energy clear. The following creative exercise can help you relate to the energy of stress within you and harness the power of your mind to clarify it, ultimately creating a peaceful internal climate.

Part One: Vision of Your Internal Climate

Sometimes it is difficult to express how our stress feels or the effect that it has on us. Long-term stress and anxiety create a climate in our minds and bodies—an inhospitable climate! Rather than using words to express your experiences, tune in to the subtle aspects of your anxiety.

1. Get a piece of paper and some crayons (or other coloring supplies), then take a few moments to breathe and become aware of your inner climate of tension. You may represent muscular tension or weakness as a tsunami, a tornado, or a barrage of rain. Perhaps there is thunder and lightning, hail, or miserable clouds. If this imagining is difficult, focus on your breath

for a moment, then ask, "If my internal state were like the weather, what kind of day would it be?"

2. Draw that internal climate as if it were a natural scene. Represent your stress or anxiety creatively: What season is it? What are the weather patterns? Are there animals here? If so, how are they reacting to the climate? Once you are finished, pause to reflect on the imagery. What are the images telling you? You may journal some ideas or share your art with a friend.
3. Next, perform a relaxation such as a body scan as described in previous exercises. Tune in to the climate this relaxation creates in your inner world, similar to the process in Step 1.
4. Repeat the expressive process for this internal climate of relaxation as in Step 2. You may choose to place this counter-image in a place you will see it frequently, such as your home office, the inside of your kitchen cupboard, or your briefcase.

Part Two: Climate Control Relaxation

Allow your imagery from the previous exercise to support this relaxation practice. This exercise calls in the power of your creative mind to unwind physical and mental stress.

1. Rest in a comfortable position. Imagine your body as a landscape. Observe the climate within, perceiving tension or stress as inclement weather systems.
2. To relax the energy of these areas, begin to imagine the weather system passing: the clouds part, the sun comes out, everything is green and blooming. Feel your body warming and unwinding as you rest in nature. Experience the stillness and quiet of a calm, comfortable space.
3. Whenever you feel stress building during your day, you may call this imagery to mind and allow it to relax and soothe you.

Mind/Body Health Through Nutrition

Food choices affect our stress levels. Comprehensive Yoga Therapy's intention is not to prescribe a specific diet; rather, its goal is to offer guidelines to examine how different kinds of food affect your specific mind-body complex. We each react differently to foods depending on our daily activity, genetics, and current stage of life.

Even throughout the course of your own life, your nutritional needs will vary. Basic principles found in yoga psychology can be very powerful in understanding nutrition from a larger point of view, even if the details about foods that aid particular health conditions are omitted. The yogic path of health examines what it means to eat for the mind by applying dietary principles versus dietary rules. From there, we can learn about some basic foods that are not medicines but simple aids to foster health and vitality.

Empty foods—those that have no vitamins, minerals, or vitality—are to be avoided. We cannot be alert and balanced when regularly eating overly processed foods such as refined sugar (including organic cane sugar, fructose, corn syrup, etc.), white flour, soft drinks, excessive caffeine, alcohol, transfats, and junk foods. It is common to resist the idea of avoiding such foods. If you simply pay attention to how you feel 10 minutes, 2 hours, or even a day after making these dietary choices, your observations—especially regarding emotions, thoughts, and stress—will speak for themselves. Once we begin to pay attention, it becomes obvious that empty foods interfere with our well-being.

Eating rich, heavy foods or even too much healthy food makes us sleepy because the body has to work so hard to process it. This leads to stress because sleepy people have trouble coping! Likewise, when we do not eat enough we may be very trim and able to think clearly, but we slowly weaken and lose our ability to maintain balance in other areas of life. Finding balance with nutrition is an important step for overall wellness and for minimizing stress, as well.

The foods we choose often mirror the state of mind. When stressed, we choose foods that create more stress such as fast food, processed carbohydrates, or sweets. When we are grounded, we cook from scratch and follow the diet we know is best for our body type. Yoga therapy does not advocate any one type of diet, aside from avoiding foods that lead to anxiousness. Instead, witness the effects your food choices have on your stress levels and shift your habits in the direction of health.

Numerous dietary approaches claim to be the best diet for healthy living. Some of the recent popular diets include vegetarianism, macrobiotics, raw food, the alkaline diet, eating for your blood type, low fat, whole food, high fat, gluten free, numerous fad "cleanses," and others. This is confusing! While most diets offer valid points, Comprehensive Yoga Therapy recommends that we educate ourselves about health and experiment with what gives each of us unique individuals optimum energy and nutrition. Factors such as activity level, metabolism, and genetic nutrient requirements all play into what makes the best nutrition plan. Consultation with a nutritionist or registered dietician may be beneficial.

Rules of Eating

Begin to shift your nutrition by following this basic principle: remain relaxed. We face so many food choices, dietary pressures, and body image issues that it is important to maintain a relaxed attitude around eating. Strict rigidity with food will worsen anxiety, especially because we eat so many times per day. Follow the 90 percent rule: eat 90 percent pure and for as long as you are not overeating. The mind is not poisoned by an imperfect diet; the mind *is* poisoned, however, by rigid beliefs. Even if the ideas in this book inspire you, incorporate the changes gradually, beginning with "Just say no to junk food." The sooner we remove these toxic "foods" from the diet, the less stressed the body will be trying to process non-food. When we make quick changes from an unhealthy to a pure diet it can be more harmful than a slow change, which would allow the body and routine to adapt.

Discover your individualized proper nutritional habits. Comprehensive Yoga Therapy avoids giving specific direction about diet or foods. As a general rule for good health consider this commonsense advice: avoid processed foods, limit your consumption of refined sugar, moderate or avoid caffeine, alcohol, white flour, soft drinks, and all junk foods. Even if you adhere to these nutritional guidelines, anxiety and stress can and usually will cause a change in weight. Notice we said "a *change* in weight," not an increase in weight or a decrease in weight. Why can't research tell us if stressed-out people will gain or lose weight? As you see throughout this book, it depends on our reaction to the stressful environment. If our habit is to eat when we get stressed then guess what: we will gain weight. If, on the other hand, our reaction is to suppress the appetite, then stress and anxiety will lead to weight loss. Strangely enough it seems as if exercise will help these opposites. If stress is making you gain weight, you will benefit from moving and burning more calories. If you are losing weight, exercise is a way to release anxious energy and stimulate the appetite (you must increase food intake in this case, otherwise exercise can lead to an undesirable accelerated weight loss). Whether or not stress affects your weight, it comes down to how you react to it!

Guidelines for Yogic Eating
• Remain relaxed. • Just say no to junk food. • Listen to your body. • Eat until satisfied, not full. • Make sure 90 percent of your diet is pure food.

Qualities of Food

Everything manifest in this world, yoga philosophy teaches, is composed of three qualities (*gunas*): pure (*sattvic*), active (*rajasic*), or dull (*tamasic*). Note that, in this case, "active" means in opposition to the desired state of stillness. Everything in the world reflects these three qualities. Our bodies and even our minds/feelings and intellects, as they are also of this world, can demonstrate these qualities. Our food choices are reflected by the effect they have on the body, life energy/breath, mind/feelings, and intellect. Review the following categories and observe the effects your nutrition choices are likely having on your state of mind. Remember to notice what happens while eating specific foods, as well as an hour afterward, throughout the day, and even how it digests through the next day.

Pure (*sattvic*) foods:

- Digest easily
- Give high nutrition
- Calm the mind
- Are not bulky or heavy

Active* (*rajasic*) foods:

- Have strong tastes
- Stimulate the senses
- Have high protein
- Feed desires

* Note that although "active" has positive connotations, in the realm of these qualities, it is synonymous with greed and agitation.

Dull (*tamasic*) foods:

- Lack nutrition
- Create a lazy and/or depressed feeling
- Are heavily processed or overcooked
- Lead to disease

Pure Foods	**Active Foods**	**Dull Foods**
Whole grains	Nuts	Refined sugar
Herbs	Cheese	Alcohol
Vegetables	Eggs	Caffeine
Fruit	Chicken	Chips, fried food
Milk	Fish	Ice cream/cookies/cake
Yogurt	Red meat	White flour
Legumes	Strong spices	Overeating/Undereating

While complete avoidance may be impossible, it is not recommended to consume dull, empty foods on a daily basis. These junk "foods" disturb body chemistry and mental state and weaken the possibility of optimal health and well-being. Once dull foods have been eliminated, the next natural step is to examine the effects of the active foods. These heavy, stimulating choices interfere with the sense of steadiness required for peace of mind. Although as a pure eater you may never eliminate active foods completely, through awareness you will clearly understand their impact on your spiritual practices and emotional balance. Thus, you may find yourself choosing legumes more often or deciding on eggs, which are less activating than animal flesh, to meet your protein needs.

A note of caution is that although pure foods will support pure living, if such a nutritional shift is done without the support of a nutritionist or dietician, the health may begin to fail, which is the worst outcome. Furthermore, a diet too low in protein will lead to erratic eating, mental distress, and sugar cravings, in addition to weakening health.

Common sense reminds us that when the mind is unbalanced on any level, food choices suffer. Imbalance occurs when we are too hungry, when breathing is stressful, emotions are distressed, the mind is distracted, or the spirit is listless. Conversely, digestion and food choices improve when we eat regularly, breathe deeply, soothe our emotions, focus the mind, and uplift the higher self.

Exercise: Mindful Eating and the Energy of Food

When we realize the effects of food on our stress and anxiety levels, we are motivated to make healthy choices. Mindful eating, or paying attention to the experience and aftereffects of eating, makes us aware. Usually we eat automatically, out of convenience and habit, and do not relate our energy levels or sense of well-being to what we have taken in. As you make different food choices, notice the effect those choices have on your energy levels and stress. Try some of the following recommendations to become more mindful of how and what you eat, and their effects on your level balance and relaxation.

1. Whenever you are feeling particularly good or particularly anxious, ask yourself, "What have I eaten in the last day?" Begin to correlate your food choices and your mood. Notice how pure food choices beget emotional balance. Likewise,

notice how unhealthy choices bring on a sense of stress, fatigue, or frustration. Let your newfound mindfulness inform your dietary needs.

2. Keep a journal of your food choices. Throughout the day, record all the foods and beverages you consume, the times, the associated emotions during eating, and the feeling after eating. You can use the chart below or find your own way of recording your meals.
3. Use the model of the layers of a person (as demonstrated in the chart below) to understand your relationship with food more deeply.
4. Use the qualities of reality to categorize your dietary choices.
5. The goal of the following food journal chart is to reveal patterns that you may not already be aware of. It helps to remain conscious of your eating habits. Try to stay focused on increased awareness and do not judge yourself for healthy or unhealthy eating habits; these will change over time. Simply do your best to record as accurately as possible and remain mindful of the effects of food on all layers of yourself. (Note: It can be challenging to discern between the mind/feelings layer and the intellect layer. Don't get too caught up in it; just do your best.)

Food/ Quality	**Breath/ Energy**	**Mind/ Feelings**	**Intellect/ Wisdom**	**Spiritual/ Higher Self**
Hamburger and soft drink Active/Dull	Rapid, shallow Low energy	Sad	Worried	Depressed
Steamed fish and veggies Active/Pure	Calm, deep Moderate energy	Happy	Clear, at peace	Optimistic

The nutrient intake from food is important for emotional balance. Some foods can indeed cause improvement in our emotional balance, but we have to be aware of dubious claims and always observe how we react to the foods we take in. Tryptophan is an amino acid that can be found in turkey, chicken, pumpkin, and some greens. It has been associated with improvements in mood, sleep, appetite, and temperature regulation among other functions. The theory is that tryptophan is converted into serotonin, through the intermediary of 5-HTP. It is very questionable if this can happen through your diet. What is more than likely needed is a purified tryptophan or 5-HTP supplements; however, there are side effects with these supplements which may be unpredictable outside of a laboratory setting. Your best bet is to enjoy a healthy diet and pay attention to how your mood shifts with your choice of a variety of foods. As you become more aware of food choices and their effects on you, you are able to plan meals in advance, choosing foods that support your mental and physical well-being. A lack of planning often leads to spur-of-the-moment, unhealthy choices, the stress of being too hungry and then bingeing, and other disruptive habits.

Allow yourself plenty of opportunity to move each day: stretch at your desk, take the stairs, park farther away from buildings. The yogic path of health teaches that movement keeps the life energy, not to mention blood and lymph, circulating and cleansed. Furthermore, we release agitation through movement, like ducks flapping their wings, dogs shaking, or teens playing football.

On the other hand, rest gives the body and mind time to integrate experiences and input through the day. Learn small cues that warn you of fatigue and intervene early. This provides quicker recovery. Reluctance to act, messiness, and isolation are often subtle hints that we are too tired. Regular rest inoculates against stress. "Doing nothing" or actively relaxing balances the breath, energy, and emotions. Resting can be done during a break at work, in a parking lot, or even standing in line!

Exercise: The 16-Point Relaxation

This exercise is an ancient yogic practice that is still very effective in the modern world. It offers focus on several vital life energy locations in the body. These vital points (*marma*) exist where there are clusters of nerve endings and therefore acute sensitivity. Below you will find the full 16-point exercise, but you may also follow an abbreviated list if you are limited for time or can't recall all of them.

1. Lie down in one of your preferred relaxation postures. Focus on each of the following areas for 10 to 30 seconds each. This practice should take 8 to 12 minutes (any longer than 12 minutes and you will likely fall asleep). Notice how your energy and subtle senses at each of these locations are different on different days. You may relate these differences to how you have been feeding yourself on all layers: body, life energy/breath, mind/feelings, intellect, and spirit/higher self.
2. Proceed with focusing on the following areas:
    - Tips of the toes
    - Ankles
    - Knees
    - Fingertips
    - Tailbone
    - Lower belly
    - Navel
    - Stomach
    - Heart
    - Throat
    - Lips
    - Tip of the nose
    - Eyes
    - Third eye
    - Forehead
    - Top of the head

Caring for your health can alleviate stress and anxiety and is one of the five paths of yoga. By feeding yourself on all layers, balancing your life energy, and being mindful of your breath and food choices, you will notice your overall energy and sense of well-being improving. Health arises through care of the whole person.

Chapter Summary

1. Our ancestors relied on herbs, food, rest, water, community, and ancient healing practices to maintain health. The comprehensive lifestyle approach of yoga revitalizes ancient methods to include physical, energetic, mental, intellectual, and spiritual health.
2. The modern world has brought great medical and technological advances, along with a lifestyle of stress and anxiety.
3. Anxious people may suffer from similar health conditions, which can often be alleviated through yoga practices.
4. We are continually taking in from the world around us; thus, nutrition for the whole person considers each layer of our beings. By shifting perceptions from the obvious to the subtle, we then apply the wise intellect to inform our responses to the ever-changing external world. This helps us be neutral, accepting, and balanced in the face of stress.
5. Food choices affect our stress levels. Correlate these effects through mindful eating and food journaling.
6. Follow these simple guidelines for eating:
    - Remain relaxed.
    - Just say no to junk food.
    - Listen to your body.
    - Eat until satisfied, not full.
    - Make sure 90 percent of your diet is pure food.
7. The boundaries between the physical body, life energy/breath, mind/feeling, intellect, and spiritual layers are permeable, and

we feed ourselves on all these levels. Through conscious direction of the breath, we can connect the five layers of our being, from the physical through the spiritual. Breath is the vehicle for life energy.

8. We each have a life energy field that surrounds us as a measurable electromagnetic field. The energetic system is usually discussed in terms of seven major energy centers or wheels (*chakras*), which can serve as a focus for yoga practice.
9. Visualization and creative expression help describe and transform the ineffable.
10. Be proactive and participatory in your personalized health plan and lifestyle.
11. Check in with your energy throughout the day to understand and purify your habits.
12. Practice the 16-point relaxation to get to know your subtle body and relax more deeply.
13. Rest more!

Now that you understand the yogic path of health, we will look at the path of work. Since most of us are required to earn a living and all of us are required to do some form of work to care for our survival, it is useful to understand work as a path to well-being. The next chapter offers yogic theory and practical recommendations to remove stress and anxiety from work life.

Chapter 8

The Yogic Path of Work

Our lives require work. Whether or not you have a job, there is the work of survival and self-care. Every day requires our efforts. The yogic path of work teaches that no matter what the task at hand, if we bring a deeper purpose, hold a spiritual attitude, and follow a prescribed, fourfold internal approach (acceptance, concentration, excellence, nonattachment), we need not ever feel stressed by our jobs.

Work Explained

Ask most people what their top three stressors are and they are sure to mention work as one of them. It would be easy to remain in a state of peace if we were able to spend our days communing with nature and others, doing yoga, eating slowly, and meditating, but that kind of life isn't a common option. When we talk about work in this chapter, we are evaluating a large percentage of your life. The average workweek is 40 hours and the average person works 50 weeks per year. That's 2,000 hours of work every year—100,000 hours (or more) over a lifetime. Plus, work from this perspective also includes housework, caring for children and aging parents, shopping, cooking, personal hygiene, and the many labors of everyday life. In reality, our activities have us working almost all the time! Thus, yoga offers clear guidelines on how to transform daily work into a path to the higher self.

Many of us separate our spiritual selves from our work life, thinking that compartmentalizing things will help us survive what can be a grueling, competitive environment. Sadly, if we split our higher selves from work, we lose a great deal of our lives to being disengaged, resentful, or anxious. Truth be told, even when we are not at work, many of us bring home the politics, stressors, and long lists, not to mention there is a great deal of work within the household; the spirit/work compartmentalization is not effective!

Ancient yogis understood that all efforts arise from a spiritual purpose or personal duty. In other words, all work is life's work; it is a path to the higher self and can be approached with reverence. The goal of this chapter is to give you simple steps to transform work into yoga practice through purpose, attitude, and the four precepts of the yogic path of work—acceptance, concentration, excellence, and nonattachment—which apply to all jobs.

Transforming Stress to Purpose

When we approach work as separate from our spiritual selves, it feels empty. There is little purpose in it beyond the fleeting material gain, which removes meaning from most of our efforts. No wonder we feel stressed, putting so much time and effort into something purposeless. When we have a personal purpose in life, we can carry it into our work throughout a lifetime. Guided by purpose, work takes on deep meaning. According to classical yoga, our purpose is divided into four arenas of duty: self, loved ones, work, and society.

Duty to Self

The primary duty is to our own health on the physical, energetic, mental, emotional, and spiritual levels. A certain level of health is required in order to accomplish most of life's tasks. The healthy person has a clear mind that can develop qualities such as faith, discipline, and compassion. When self-care is practiced, we develop strength from within. This is not the same as selfishness. Spiritual purpose views self-care through a broader lens. For example, some people frequently call in sick when they "don't feel like working." They may cite self-care as the reason for this; however, when viewed through the lens of purpose, we do not shirk our responsibilities in the interest of caring for ourselves. Rather, we evaluate the whole situation: "Why do I often not feel like it? How are my energy levels? My nutrition? My emotions?" From an enquiry into the entire situation surrounding the need for self-care, we can take direct action to improve our overall situation, rather than relying on habitual, disruptive, short-term solutions. Addressing issues at their roots gives understanding to all our levels of need and is the proper realization of this primary purpose. *Duty to self relates to the higher self*, our spiritual development and personal health. Learn to nurture your spirit with self-understanding. When we are healthy and at peace, we are empowered to share that peace with others. Taking care of ourselves, when done for the benefit of others, is virtuous.

Duty to Loved Ones

The second spiritual priority is to our loved ones. It is important to feel at peace with interpersonal relationships. While each person's family situation is different, we all have roles to play with our loved ones. Due to the complexity of loving relationships, it can be difficult to figure out how to express interpersonal responsibilities in a healthy fashion, without becoming distant, enabling, or codependent. Discussing healthy relationships with a yoga therapist, counselor, or like-minded friends may help define the boundaries of relational responsibilities.

Duty to Work and Duty to Society

The same approach can be taken to the third and fourth priorities: work and our role in society. Before contributing to society in general, it is prudent to have good health, strong relationships, and steady work. Once we are able to maintain a healthy spiritual growth routine, have balanced relationships, and hold a job, community service is important. Not only do we have a moral duty to contribute to society, but life has more meaning when we contribute to something greater than ourselves. Find a cause that is important to you and engage in making things better.

Of course, we do not actually follow these four areas of purpose in a step-by-step fashion. The priorities help us structure life through awareness and intentionality. The highest level of purpose is to see each endeavor from a spiritual perspective. For example, taking out the compost may be viewed as an act of spiritual growth, caring for the family, a worthy job, or environmental action. If we make the compost an exercise of service, we feel full of care amidst the aromatic vegetation. The job is uplifting when viewed in the light of purpose. This approach aligns your work with the first priority of self-care by offering spiritual fulfillment through a purposeful intention.

Exercise: Your Mind at Work

Take a moment to examine your own attitude toward work. Give yourself the freedom to answer truthfully and without judgment, even if your answers are not what you think you should be or even what you know intellectually to be true. We are seeking the answers that hide in the back of the mind, so do not edit yourself. This exercise helps you get in touch with your automatic response to the idea of work. This may give you insights about your underlying beliefs that contribute to work stress.

1. First, reflect on work in general, be it your household chores, current and past jobs, or the first things that come to mind when considering work. Notice what happens in your body as you think of work. How is your breath? What is happening in your muscles? How is your heartbeat? Do you notice a sense of strength, weakness, tension, relaxation, pain, ease…?
2. As you continue to think about work in general, move your awareness to a deeper layer. Notice your state of mind, emotions, and quality of thoughts. What feelings do you have? Are memories arising? Do you hear phrases repeating themselves? Do old scripts come to mind?

True Purpose in Action

The yogic path of work requires us to take action in our lives. This action arises from our personal purpose of spiritual growth and connection to the higher self. Rather than seeking fulfillment from a particular job, we come to experience fulfillment through our relationship with work itself. Within the work, we discover inner peace as we explore life's lessons. This approach allows our ultimate purpose to be practiced now, wherever we are.

Awareness of our life's purpose starts with recognizing that being a loving, compassionate, accepting, forgiving, or otherwise spiritual person is at its heart. From this core understanding of purpose we can harness our talents and behave in ways that increase our expressions of virtue. In some ways, it is a great relief to know that our spiritual purpose can be revealed in the midst of ordinary tasks.

We can view our work from the inner lesson that we are striving to learn. We are able to fill our hearts with love while doing accounting (care for loved ones' or clients' finances) or while tending our children (self-realization through bonding). As we hone our natural talents and behaviors, we increase the expression of purpose in life. This is a service to ourselves and others.

Working in this purposeful way brings a deep quality to everyday tasks. Our purpose thrives in the spirit with which we perform each task, rendering the task itself nearly irrelevant. Work is no longer stress or a burden, and it is impossible to be anxious while engaging in spiritual action. Work is often difficult and stressful when the attitude is not focused on spiritual growth. However, even a mundane job may turn into the means for lasting happiness. This purpose permeates all moments; experience work for enlightenment. Our true purpose is the spirit with which we perform actions, rather than the actions themselves.

Exercise: Feel the Action You Perform

We tend to think of a task as the job itself. In the previous section you learned to see your work as part of your personal purpose and a path to spiritual growth. Now the task is not the work itself but staying connected to its underlying purpose (some form of connection with the higher self). When we approach a task with clear purpose, we experience the task with clarity and purposefulness.

1. Identify the purpose, or spiritual lesson, of your current life's intention. This purpose supports you in feeling the action. To discover a purpose, you may revisit your intention for reading this book or call to mind an aspect of yourself you are working on at this time. Your purpose may be a specific spiritual lesson or perhaps it is an internal habit you are trying to change. Your purpose is your own; trust yourself with whatever you come up with. You can refine it as time goes on.
2. Think of an everyday job that creates stress. It may be a household chore, one of your duties at work, or another common task. Notice the patterned thoughts and feelings that go along with this job.
3. Smile as you bring your purpose to mind. Begin *feeling* your personal purpose. Continue turning up the corners of the mouth and softening the eyes as you hold the purpose, virtue, or intention with you. At the same time, bring to mind the stressful task. Experience, through your imagination, how you can do the task and feel very purposeful and spiritually uplifted.
4. If possible, perform this or another stressful task now, keeping the smile and purposeful state of mind with you. Notice that the anxiety is minimized in the face of your purpose and sense of higher self. We feel the action we perform.

The outcomes of the previous exercise demonstrate a key concept of Comprehensive Yoga Therapy: "Healing begins in the mind." You recover from anxiety and remove stress by changing your inner environment. Stress transformation happens not only through outward action, but through the internal choices we make. Internal action involves understanding the intention that spurs the action in the first place.

When a spiritual intention guides our action, in this case our work, we are immediately set into a different state of mind. The yogic path of work brings us into a higher state of consciousness on the job. Rather than compartmentalizing spirituality and work, we experience a personal unity through all of our actions. Our jobs, be they paid work or household chores, are transformed into times to cultivate a spiritual attitude. This attitude then soothes the nervous system and empowers the psyche. Work becomes yoga practice!

The Stress of Technology

For many of us, "working" means interacting with technology. Over the course of just a few decades, our lives have become immersed in electronics. Children spend the bulk of their playtime indoors, interacting with screens and controllers. Even adults have taken on hobbies in front of blue screens, spending less time connecting with each other in genuine and supportive ways. It is easier to comment on a social media website than to reach out and show genuine support. Why is that? The research on why we act differently on social media than face-to-face is in its early stages. One aspect might be that on social media we can act without having a real person in front of us. We can be the king in our kingdom—that is, until someone shoots down our "well thought out" opinions. Social media allows us some disguise and distance.

In a lot of ways, the social media issue is a matter of return on investment. It takes more energy to reach out to someone in person rather than virtually. To really feel compassionate connection, your own neurons must fire in a similar way to the emotion that you want the person you are reaching out to feel. If you are not capable of feeling an emotion of caring or empathy, then seeing the face of the person you are reaching out to might be confusing and frightening. Your mirror neurons do not know what the other person is feeling, and you cannot genuinely reach out, and the person you are reaching out to might sense that, and you will be seen as a fraud, and… Oh, it is so much safer to reach out on social media to say "I am thinking about you," since our mirror neurons are not required to fire then—and we can eat while we are typing. Technology has become our recreation and social time!

Technology's role in the workplace has extended many people's workdays to eighteen hours or more. We are always "on"—reachable by anyone anywhere through mobile phones, which also receive email. Many middle managers receive correspondence at 8PM from bosses who expect an immediate request be completed by 9AM the next day! Ultimately, this limits our sense of personal safety as we have little escape from the demands of our work life and the twenty-four-hour accessibility of technology. Perhaps you are aware of ways that technology is contributing to stress, anxiety, and isolation in your own life.

Exercise: Assessing the Truth About Technology

This exercise offers you the chance to explore your relationship with technology and the effect it is having on your human relationships, work stress, and anxiety levels. Answer the questions honestly; you are the only one who needs to know.

1. How many hours per day do you engage with technology? Calculate the time you spend surfing the Internet, watching TV, reading e-books, playing video games, and using a smartphone. Because we tend to underestimate the amount of time we spend on technology, try creating a log for a few days to gain a truthful perception.
2. This step requires you to take a break from technology. This can be as short as an hour once you return home from work or as long as a weekend where you do a "technology fast" and do not turn on a computer, phone, television, or radio. After a period of time without technology, practice a body scan as described in Chapter 4. Notice how easy it is to relax and what your usually tense places feel like. Journal about what you notice.

3. After you have engaged with technology again, do another body scan. Pay special attention to your eyes, shoulders, neck, and any other areas of the body that draw your awareness. Journal these observations.
4. What did you do before technology was so prevalent? Make a list of activities you enjoyed that did not involve electricity, blue screens, and remote controls.

Technology and the Nervous System

Research continues on the effects technology has on our health. Blue screens are notorious for disrupting our sleep patterns. There is evidence that our breath becomes more rapid and shallow from so much time in office chairs. Gazing at tiny screens requires the action of the cone cells in our eyes and dilation of our pupils; this is also how the eyes engage when we are in fight-flight-or-freeze mode. When we watch television, our brain waves are similar to those when we are asleep, which leaves us highly hypnotizable to the barrage of fearful and sexual imagery. This in turn activates our base survival instincts, which steers us further from our spiritual selves. Furthermore, studies have shown that when we see someone else in pain, our own brains light up as if it had happened to us. Nightly news engages this empathy without our knowing, and part of us can go to bed feeling as if we ourselves were at war and victims of recent violence.

All the above activities and so many others that involve technology actually change our brain. Studies in children indicate that the more they use technology the more likely they are to be depressed. We know that depression inhibits certain areas of the brain, and that organs (including the brain) become very good at doing what they do a lot of. If we keep inhibiting certain areas of the brain they will not develop. If we develop certain areas, such as the area that is related to anxiety, through constantly playing violent or fast-paced computer games or watching violent newscasts, then the area of the brain related to anxiety will strengthen. Once an area of the brain has increased or decreased in size it becomes more difficult to change it back to balance. This is similar to muscles. The muscles we use a lot will become strong and others will weaken. If we continue in that strengthening pattern we will eventually develop a musculoskeletal imbalance and, in time, an injury. Now with the use of brain scans we can see that technology can develop nervous system/brain imbalance, especially in a developing brain. Since brains continue to develop throughout life that means the nervous system/brain imbalance can develop in all of us, which makes us all susceptible to problems with stress and anxiety. The good news is it also means we can develop nervous system and brain balance for peace!

Now that you are aware of the effects of technology on your physical health, you can remind yourself that much of your everyday stress may be induced by it! The next time you become anxious, take a break from the technology. Just one minute of standing, stretching, or eyes-closed deep breathing can begin to regulate the nervous system and set you back into the peaceful rest-and-digest mode.

Unplugging and Other Recommendations

Remember when email was becoming mainstream? We were told that things could be done so much more quickly that we would have more leisure time. In fact, if every company started using email, we could be so productive during our workweeks that we would soon be enjoying three-day weekends as the norm! Looking at our lives years later, we see that the opposite is true. Impatience is rampant and things move so quickly that on-the-job immediacy is an assumed requirement. We may feel as if we are constantly running, and that pace is stressful.

To help soothe anxiety levels, every so often commit to unplugging. If you can, take a week out of every season and stay away from blue screens, devices, and information overload. If your job involves technology, try to limit it by saving up non-tech tasks and completing them during your "unplugged" retreat. You will be amazed by the effect this has on your sleep, well-being, creativity, and even weight!

There is a saying: "You can't unring a bell." Well, you can't unplug the blue screen, either. Not most people and not forever, anyway. Nonetheless, when we are aware of the insidious damage technology can cause, we are empowered to shift our habits. Even small changes like turning off devices an hour before bed or only checking email at certain hours of the day can go a long way in reducing our anxiety and improving health. Remember that the anxiety you feel throughout the day may be triggered by physiological responses to technology, not actual fearsome things in life. Finally, you are not required to stay apprised of global details. Take a break from the news, knowing that global and political trends will continue without your constant monitoring. Although technology has helped us in many ways, it comes with its detriments and it is beneficial to unplug on a regular basis.

Spiritual Attitude of Work

Most of us do not consider work as part of spirituality. However, we experience an internal disconnection when we compartmentalize work from the rest of our lives. Yoga (union) reminds us that connection is an essential part of well-being; it is no wonder that we become anxious when we separate out such an integral part of our everyday lives. It is possible to find the higher self in our work life and unite with our sense of spirit at work every day. By cultivating a spiritual attitude, we are able to connect more deeply to our lives—even the parts that seem to cause stress—and live more fully.

Ask the average person how work is going and they are likely to complain about the burden of it all. The socially accepted response is to commiserate, finding our own disgruntlement and sharing it. This creates a kind of "groupthink" of pain, where most of us expect our jobs to be frustrating, stressful, and upsetting not only in terms of the duties, but also the politics of hierarchy and interpersonal relationships. Assuming that work is stressful on many levels creates a state of mind that contributes to stress.

In yoga therapy sessions, it is common to see clients who are anxious about the long hours, task overload, and constant threat of downsizing. Deep breathing and relaxation techniques are important interventions to balance the nervous system and create an internal climate of relaxation; however, these techniques have minimal impact if the mind is stressed. A profound shift in anxiety can occur when the attitude toward work changes.

Likes, Expectations, Desires

The main problems in our attitude toward work tend to be unconscious. Likes (and dislikes!), expectations, and desires are programmed into us over years of socialization and media influence. These barriers to well-being combine in our psyche, coloring our work activities and forming attitudes of judgment and hierarchy rather than equanimity and balance. Likes, expectations, and desires express themselves as a general resistance to certain aspects of our work lives. Once they are understood, they lose their power to create anxiety.

Likes and dislikes, in their healthy form, are simply expressions of our aptitudes. We have an affinity to what we are interested in and skilled at. In early childhood, our higher selves shone through the games and activities we enjoyed, and there was no developed sense of like and dislike. For example, if you loved building blocks you may have the natural disposition to become an architect or carpenter, while if you enjoyed books you may have the innate talent to be a professor or editor. Affinities teach us about ourselves and do not typically create stress.

Eventually, our childhood affinities and aversions became categorized. We learned to form likes and dislikes for every imaginable part of life, from games to food to friends. The like / dislike stage is a necessary part of discerning moral development. The problem is that this stage of thinking did not progress beyond a state of mere judgment. Most of our everyday likes and dislikes have very little to do with morality and a great deal to do with comfort. Ironically, our wish to avoid external things that cause discomfort creates the internal discomfort of stress!

Yoga philosophy teaches us not to take life so personally; we are free from the stress of not liking something. Instead, we may cultivate an attitude of acceptance of the inevitable and let things be as they are. We no longer need to feel anxious because the office changed its reporting format, our children wear too much black, or we have to learn new computer software. This is not to say that you will be lazy when it is appropriate to take action; rather, you will not rail against that which is unchangeable. Letting go of personal likes and dislikes removes their stress and frees the mind to experience life as it is.

Expectations lead to immediate unhappiness because almost nothing in life goes according to our version of reality. We may expect work to be one way and in reality it is better or worse than that. How the job actually is externally is beyond our control. Even if we had a sense of what to expect at some point, people and the environment are shifting on a daily basis. Everything around us is constantly changing and sometimes our expectations are not aligned with this simple truth. Expectations are programmed over years of patterning, perception, and internal dialogue; they may be unconscious. Remember the adage "Expectations are planned disappointments." Our personal stories of what we expect from reality can make us anxious—we know on some level that expectations are rarely realized. With awareness of our preconceived ideas, it is possible to shift these expectations into a neutral observance of reality, which in turn neutralizes our stress.

Desires are slightly different than expectations. Where expectations are about our judgments of how things should be, desires are what we hope for. They are rooted deep in the psyche and are not so easily uprooted, understood, or transformed. Desires stem from beliefs and goals that are dear to us. They can be strong enough to make us endure hardships in order to reach a goal. They may be noticed and understood but actually shifting our desires is a longer process that takes awareness, time, and a lot of diligent self-study. The outcomes of our desires and work may not meet our expectations, either. When our primary desire is union with the higher self, or enlightenment, we are freed from the anxiety of likes, dislikes, expectations, and lower desires.

Exercise: Digging at the Roots of Work Stress

We often assume that work is meant to be stressful—why else would so many people be stressed by work? However, as we discussed in Part I, our underlying beliefs create a great deal of unnecessary stress. This exercise examines the roots of your work stress. By digging at these roots, you may be able to weed them out completely and enjoy greater relaxation with your responsibilities.

1. List ten of the major tasks you perform on a daily basis. Note your likes/dislikes of the activity, your expectations around it, and your desires. Do not self-correct, judge, or write what you think you should say; just be honest and notice your raw feelings toward the activities. The following examples show you how you might complete this exercise in your own way.

Task 1: Doing the Dishes

The dishes are driving me crazy. The kids don't carry the dishes to the kitchen and after a long day at work, I have to do chores until bedtime. I am resenting the dishes and my family because there's just not enough time for me. I dislike being busy. I expect people to clean their own dishes and they don't. I want them to love me and am afraid to ask for help. I want more restful time and for others to do their share!

Task 2: Returning Emails

- Like: Nice to be in touch with some of these people; efficient way of communicating
- Dislike: Filtering through junk; emails that require me to do more work
- Unconscious expectation: Maybe I won't get so many emails
- Conscious expectation: Email is now a part of life; email should be quick and easy
- Desire: Stay employed; keep in touch with people

2. The intention of this exercise is to gain understanding of underlying attitudes that cause stress. Now that you have explored the thoughts and feelings associated with your daily work, you can see how these (dis)likes, expectations, and desires create an internal climate of anxiety around everyday tasks. To counter this effect and deconstruct those old attitudinal habits, compose a brief affirmation or prayer. For the next three weeks, read it at the beginning of your day, and anytime you feel stressed or anxious, or feel like unhealthy beliefs are arising. Re-

main aware of the effect your prayer/affirmation has on your stress levels and general reaction to work.

Task 1: Affirmation for Doing the Dishes
I nurture myself by nurturing home. Doing the dishes with the family is time for connection.

Task 2: Affirmation for Returning Emails
May my higher self guide my words and responses to all work.

By changing our beliefs and gut reactions to our responsibilities, we set the stage for a more peaceful, healthy relationship with work. As we persist in cultivating a spiritual attitude about our duties, the entire job becomes colored with ease and freedom from stress.

Students of yoga come to understand that the ultimate purpose in life is connection to the higher self. Because yoga is nondogmatic, it does not define what the higher self is or a singular path to realize it. Rather, yoga offers a technology of philosophy and practice that guides us to internal understanding and deep faith. This is our ultimate purpose.

Each of us innately identifies our purpose through what we love, appreciate, and are interested in. Our personal aptitudes, individual gifts and strengths, as well as our natural enthusiasm lead us to an understanding of our higher self. We know we are living in alignment with our purpose when we feel authentic, calm, caring, and free from anxiety. Spiritual life is guided by this alignment with personal purpose. Our highest duty in life is to explore what this means to us as individuals and endeavor, through action, word, and especially thought, to align with who we really are. This unending quest is spiritual growth.

No matter what our work is, we can bring this personal purpose into it. To the objective viewer, there is very little difference between someone begrudgingly sweeping the floor and someone who is doing the job for their enlightenment. The state of mind between these two sweepers, however, are worlds apart.

Where one is focusing on and, indeed, cultivating misery, the other senses a spiritual intention in even this simple task, and is able to align all everyday efforts with an ultimate purpose.

The Fourfold Path

The yogic path of work teaches us that all actions—from washing the dishes to closing million-dollar deals—are spiritual opportunities. When we remember our personal purpose while working, we are uplifted by any task. On the other hand, if we perform the work without the perspective of a higher purpose we feel burdened and stressed. Yoga philosophy offers a fourfold approach to work to keep us connected to spiritual purpose. By following the fourfold approach, we are able to complete any task with ease and peace of mind, be it at home, at work, or even within ourselves. The fourfold yoga philosophy of work is:

- Acceptance
- Concentration
- Excellence
- Nonattachment

This approach offers us a process for removing the burden of stress by keeping our internal purpose vital and top-of-mind throughout the process of work.

Acceptance

The first precept of this fourfold method is to cultivate acceptance for the task at hand. This sounds simple enough, but being fully accepting is actually a difficult and uncommon thing. Our cultural norms and typically self-centered approach to life create internal barriers to acceptance. When we identify those barriers, they can no longer silently sabotage our tranquility. Furthermore, as we cultivate awareness of our mental habits, we begin to notice that our initial reactions to most daily requirements involve some form of resistance or negativity. There is a process for transforming all of these stressful habits into equanimity and acceptance.

Yoga teaches that all actions are neutral. This point is illustrated by asking any given group, "Who here likes decorating?" All the homey, creative people raise their hands and tell you about their connection to color, beautifying their living space, and the satisfaction of having their environment reflect their inner selves. Others in the room will grumble at the labor of painting, selecting knick-knacks, and fussing over arrangements. The same task is met differently by different minds. This is due in part to personal disposition as well as judgments and beliefs. The first step of the fourfold path, acceptance, reminds us that although the human mind creates attachment and stress, all jobs in and of themselves are neutral.

Concentration

Whereas an absence of acceptance makes the mind jumpy and resistant, when our minds are set in neutral acceptance it is easier to focus on work. Concentration occurs when we focus body and mind on one task without distraction; work can be a meditation. It is easy to describe concentration but very difficult to achieve. Concentration requires continual effort over a long period of time and needs dedication to stay focused and limit distractions. A special amount of patience is required in the work environment, which offers a multitude of interruptions and distractions.

The trick to mastering concentration is the ability to return to the present moment whenever we are distracted. This is a discipline. Practice can start by simply being present with each breath. It does not matter how many times you get distracted, just stay committed to coming back to the present breath as soon as you notice your mind wander off. It *will* wander off, again and again, for the rest of your life. That's okay. What's important isn't that it wanders; what's important is bringing it back. There are many training tools for concentration, such as repeating a silent prayer or mantra, sensing body movements, and proactively eliminating distractions.

Distractions come in many forms, including but not limited to habits (staying up too late, substance use, gaming), emotions (dislike, worry, fear, pressure), relationships (coworker politics, family problems), or intentions (not having one, being selfishly motivated). Most profoundly, we lose concentration because we get worried about what will happen once the task is done. We often feel the most distracted at a new job or one we do not have aptitudes for because we fear it will not be good enough. The reality is not everyone can be good at everything. Adjusting our habits, attitudes, beliefs, and intentions can vastly improve concentration.

Exercise: Awareness at Work

A frequent theme in this book is the importance of mental awareness. Our patterned thoughts and beliefs go a long way in determining our levels of stress or relaxation. By applying the principle of concentration, we can bring focus to our daily tasks and imbue them with a sense of well-being, gradually replacing stress and anxiety with uplifting feelings. This exercise gives you concrete steps on how to do so.

1. During an average workday this week, observe where your mind goes when you lose concentration. Pick a cue to remind you to notice, such as every time a phone rings or you change tasks. Jot down the specific thoughts and feelings that disrupt your concentration throughout the day. If possible, have a journal with you; otherwise, even scraps of paper will do—you can bring them home and paste them into your journal. What's most important is getting the thoughts down in a few words while they are still fresh.
2. Soon a pattern will arise offering you greater understanding about the underlying anxieties that draw you away from concentration and empower you to make shifts in your beliefs and habits.

3. While learning the skill of concentration, do not be disturbed or upset when you get distracted; instead, work on practicing the first precept of this approach, acceptance. Continue returning to the present experience and remain resolved to learn about yourself. Eventually, we all see progress in our concentration skills.

As you focus on one task, and leave the rest to a larger reality, you will develop faith. The practice of concentration strengthens our ability to trust in a larger process, which in turn reduces stress.

Excellence

Excellence is the third precept of the fourfold path in the yogic path of work. In this philosophy, excellence can relate to the external product of work but more importantly it relates to *internal* excellence. External excellence is demonstrated by a job well done; internal excellence is a sincere endeavor to do our best. We know what it is like to go through the motions of a job without care—it is not fulfilling, even if it turns out well. We have also experienced doing our best and having it turn out poorly. Ironically, this usually feels better than the former situation. There is something inherently rewarding about giving a task our all. It is a concentrated, connecting experience and is the epitome of internal excellence.

It can take a lifetime to strike a balance between excellence in the mind and external performance. Tipping the balance too much to either side of the equation results in less efficiency. If we are obsessed with maintaining peace of mind at work, we may become lazy or unproductive. If we feel pressured to do a great job, we may sacrifice our health or personal relationships. In the end, both an internal peace of mind and a high level of performance are needed to have lasting fulfillment in work.

Remember that there is a difference between excellence and perfectionism! It is impossible to do better than our best. Nothing natural is perfect, except in its own way. The same is true for each of us and the results of our labor. Earlier, we discussed that "You feel the action you perform." When dedicated to excellence in an endeavor, you feel excellent in the moment. This aligns with the previous precepts of acceptance and concentration. The end result of your labors is not relevant to the *experience* of doing your best; when you offer excellence, you have fully given of yourself. Even more, you feel excellent!

When the concept of excellence is applied to daily life, every task can help improve the body-mind health. Excellence in paying bills is a pleasant attitude of appreciation for the service received. Writing clearly on checks and envelopes are also ways to practice excellence. Washing clothes and dishes well, being polite to strangers in public, and waiting patiently at the traffic light are examples of maintaining an excellent state of mind while performing a simple, everyday action. From this perspective, excellence can encompass everything we do in daily life.

Nonattachment

Nonattachment is key to a stress-free life. By practicing the fourth precept, nonattachment, we can be at peace in every situation. The nonattached worker views work as a path of spiritual growth; thus, work becomes a privilege rather than a burden. Every task is an opportunity to learn, grow, and elevate ourselves beyond the attachments of life. The previous three precepts relate to this: being thankful for work elevates our acceptance, spiritual attitude helps hold our concentration, and commitment to excellence is cleansing for the soul.

For example, we wash dishes to wash dishes. We are not attached to getting it done quickly, or how dirty the dishes are, or how many in the stack are actually ours; we simply wash dishes. Every resistance to working with a selfless attitude can be observed throughout the process of washing. An attached worker is irritated when someone brings more dirty dishes after the washing is complete. The dishwasher has a chance to learn a life lesson in letting go of the irritation while performing a daily chore.

We have been conditioned through desserts after supper, grades in school, and raises at work to expect rewards for jobs well done. The work itself becomes less important than the effects of the work. The yogic path of work reminds us that the greatest, most sustained rewards are internal. In truth, the only thing we have control over is our internal state and our efforts. When we concentrate on what matters and do our best, we can detach from the rest.

Another definition of nonattachment is surrendering the fruits of our action to a larger reality (God, Creator, the universe). It helps to remember that no job is done by a single person. Even in washing the dishes, there are whole teams of people who made the soap, purified and transported the water, created the heating systems, and so on. The water is given from the earth and clouds. Furthermore, most of our jobs were not invented by us. We are standing on the shoulders of all those who figured out these ever more efficient ways of completing tasks. In practicing nonattachment, we might thank the Higher Reality for being healthy enough to wash the dishes! The attached person takes credit for the work; the nonattached person perceives the divine processes at work.

The fourfold approach to work begins with acceptance of any situation considering how it fits into the larger reality. Full concentration is applied to the task, absorbing us in the work as a meditation. Through this focus, our best efforts arise. Excellence relates to state of mind while working, as well as job performance. Lastly, we remain nonattached to the results of work. Nonattachment reminds us to enjoy the job for its own sake and not for the end results. Since we typically cannot control what happens with our work once it is out of our hands, we do not need to carry stress about the end results.

Exercise: The Fourfold Yogic Path of Work and You

We accept that some tasks disrupt our peace of mind. Ultimately, however, this disruption is what contributes to our stress and anxiety. A task is just a task and our beliefs make it stressful, enjoyable, icky, and so on. The following exercise helps you take the feelings of work you like and apply them to those you don't. It may take practice, but learning this skill can save you years of stress!

1. Jot down a task you enjoy. How do you apply acceptance, concentration, excellence, and nonattachment to that task?
2. Now think of a task that causes you stress. Describe how you can apply each of these precepts to it as well.
3. How can you apply the fourfold approach to work more clearly? What is important to remember? Is there an affirmation you can use? How can you keep these precepts with you while performing more challenging work?

Free yourself from the stress of resistance by accepting your work. Then the joy of working, as well as mental practice, allows complete concentration. Excellence includes an inner state of peace as well as an external mastery of the task. By doing your best in the moment, you become nonattached to the end result and are at peace with any outcome.

Taking Control of Your Work Stress

Who is in charge of your life? Who decides how you respond to responsibilities and stressors? Sometimes anxiety makes us feel like we are out of control, as if we were not in charge of our internal or external worlds. By setting an intention, reducing extraneous demands, understanding our personal purpose, and following the fourfold approach to work, we are able to gain mastery over our own stress and environment.

Through the fourfold yogic process of work, we choose to respond to life on our own terms while continuing to meet our responsibilities. External behavior is in line with who we know we are inside while that internal self is completely free. We let go of "should" and "have to," deciding instead to perceive our choice and purpose behind all tasks. It is not always easy or fun, but because we approach each situation with a yogic mindset, we can use the techniques of this chapter to transform our reactions and choose freedom from stress at every step.

Exercise: Purpose and the Fourfold Yogic Path of Work

This exercise gives you a summary of this chapter and something concrete to keep with you as you continue working toward a stress-free approach to your responsibilities.

1. Considering all you have learned in this chapter, what is your current spiritual intention? It may be "To accept myself even when I am not perfect" or "To remain relaxed during tasks I dislike" or "To smile and focus while I wash dishes." Be as specific as possible, noticing how you feel in your body and the thoughts that arise when you focus on it.
2. Combine this intention with your intention for removing stress/anxiety. Hold this intention as a deep spiritual purpose and carry it with you through your workday. Each evening, record how this intention helped you lessen anxiety.

As you apply the lessons from this chapter to your work life, you will begin to reduce your anxiety and find pockets of the day where you cultivate a higher level of internal harmony. Have patience with yourself and, in time, the moments where you experience the freedom of nonattachment will expand. Remember that it is a process to transform work into an internal yoga practice. Living a spiritual life takes ongoing commitment to that highest duty of self-care; if we are going to remove anxiety, these techniques are not something to be tried once and forgotten. Patience, nonattachment to the results, and ongoing practice are important. Cultivating peace of mind and confidence at work keeps even the most mundane routine full of wonder.

The approach to the yogic path of work includes an inward as well as outward focus. Understand that this path is to be of service, first to self, then to loved ones, work, and society. By gaining inner knowledge, you become able to work with efficiency and grace, improving stress levels and external performance. Personal purpose guides work. The fourfold path cultivates the highest integrity through acceptance, concentration, excellence, and nonattachment to the results. In turn, all of these shifts create an internal climate of relaxation and faith. When we continue with the path of work, our jobs become a gift to our enlightenment. Tasks take on a reverent quality: work as worship.

Chapter Summary

1. Work, including our efforts for the body and home, may be the main cause of modern stress. Bringing spirituality into our efforts replaces stressful feelings.
2. Connect work to a spiritual sense of purpose.
3. Follow your spiritual priorities, as follows: higher self, loved ones, work, society.
4. We feel the action we perform. Have a personal intention to explore through your relationship to work. Thus, fulfillment doesn't come from finishing a job, but rather, the quality brought to it.
5. Electronics amplify stress; unplug often.
6. The roots of stress in the mind are likes, dislikes, desires, and expectations.
7. The fourfold yoga philosophy of work is:
    - Acceptance
    - Concentration
    - Excellence
    - Nonattachment
8. Internal purpose throughout the process of work limits the stressful effects of external situations and outcomes.

Where this chapter focused on work life and your relationship with tasks, the next chapter focuses on your emotional life and interpersonal relationships. We will look at relationships with yourself as well as others and the Divine (however you define that). Research indicates that relationships are the main source of our stress; the following is an important chapter.

Chapter 9

The Yogic Path of Relationships and Emotions

Even the most fulfilling relationships can be stressful at times. In this chapter we enquire about how our emotions are expressed through our bodies and what you can do to listen more deeply. We look at how your relationship with yourself informs all other relationships. This chapter examines how to stay relaxed when dealing with others through boundaries and communication skills and how a relationship with the Divine keeps our emotions uplifted and calm.

What Is the Yogic Path of Relationships and Emotions?

Most of the life events psychologists consider most stressful concern relationships: to loved ones, living places, career, and health. It's no surprise that the death of or separation from loved ones are considered highly stressful but even taking a vacation is on the list, which shows how sensitive we are to any change in our relationship with reality! Think of how much stress you have in relationships with others or when your routine changes, as well as the amount of joy you may receive from loving relationships.

Yoga therapy is effective in helping people manage the emotional nature of relationships. Emotions and health are linked: the psychosomatic reality. An upset stomach commonly relates to worry that binds the vagus nerve complex linking the brain and guts. A heavy heart brings the shoulders forward in times of sadness, leading to shortness of breath, back pain, and possibly chest pain. Irritants that we name "a pain in the neck" indicate an underlying psychological state of imbalance. Unlike acute medical pains and diseases, psychosomatic imbalances tend to appear in more subtle or changing ways. However, what begins as subtle levels of stress in the body and mind may lead to anxiety and other health conditions. Yoga therapy helps balance emotions, health, and relationships.

Exercise: Your Psychosomatic Tendencies

It is beneficial to know how your body reacts to emotional stress. The body often gives us cues to change things before we are consciously aware that anxiety is building. By identifying your psychosomatic tendencies, you can be more awakened to taking action when these symptoms arise and de-stress yourself.

1. Are you aware of any of the following psychosomatic symptoms? Have you experienced them in the past? Check the symptoms in this list that relate to your experiences—you are not alone if you check every box!

√	Psychosomatic Symptom
	Shortness of breath
	Poor sleep
	Stomachache
	Headache
	Constipation / diarrhea
	Tight jaw / clenched teeth / temporomandibular joint (TMJ) issues
	Kinked neck / hunched shoulders
	Racing heart / arrhythmia / chest pains
	Dizziness / vertigo
	Lower back pain
	Other:

2. Alongside each box that you checked, note one thing you can do to soothe the physical responses to your stress. For example, if you experience shortness of breath, you might try a prolonged exhale. If you experience a kinked neck or shoulders, you can do basic yoga postures to loosen the musculature.

Compared to the vast amount of research on physical ailments, little has been proven about the physical effects of psychosomatic illnesses. However, everyone knows that strong, uncomfortable emotional states such as sadness, anger, and worry lead to anxiety, depression, and other mental health issues. This may be true in subtle ways, as well. The effects of strong emotional states on physical health have only been formally researched in recent years, but much has been proven or at least suggested during the short time that this kind of research has been conducted.

Among the most solid research findings are depression's impact on physical health and wellness. Depression slows down our ability to heal from physical illness. Close emotional and social connections tend to lead to longer and healthier lives, while suppressed emotions and lack of closeness tend to lead to a suppressed immune system and increased mortality. So research is finally catching up to something we have always known: our relationships are important for our health.

Relationship to Your Self

Dedicated yoga practitioners who live in mountain monastic settings are often revered as highly evolved spiritual beings and are considered to be free from material desires; however, they still have to deal with each other! Monks have internal tools to cope with the stresses that naturally occur when different people come together. Culturally, it is acceptable for us to complain about and blame others for our feelings, which denies personal responsibility and power over the emotional response. There is always opportunity to relate relationship difficulties to our own spiritual lessons. Naturally, there will be times that no amount of intentionality can keep us from getting hurt. This is when we must remember the fundamental attitude of being a student of life. We can learn and grow from our reactions to others. This internal inquiry is the difference between the monks and the average, reactive person still driven by external circumstances.

There is very little self-mastery when the external experiences dictate the internal state. If someone smiles or shows you love, then you may feel loved. If they are rude, you may feel hurt. Usually the external experiences trigger something that is already active within us. In this dynamic, you see that what we resist persists. In other words, a quality that bothers us about others is usually something that we are fighting within ourselves. If we don't rectify the internal quality, accepting ourselves and endeavoring to transform the unwanted quality into a strength, we continue to see it reflected in others and remain upset by it. Through this process of acceptance, we connect to the higher self through relationship challenges.

The higher self shines through when we define ourselves from the inside out. If we decide to be peaceful, when someone is kind we respond with compassion and peace, and when someone is rude we respond with compassion and peace. We do not have to be pulled away from the higher self into rudeness. Once determined to be a peaceful person, the external need not dictate the internal state.

According to classical yoga philosophy, the primary purpose in life is to connect to the higher self. This colors our responsibilities to loved ones, work, and society. Neglecting the fundamental duty of spiritual self-care leads to stress and anxiety. Some typical examples of this personal neglect are overworking, eating poorly, not resting sufficiently, not exercising enough, or emotionally neglecting our families. When we integrate the fundamental purpose of connecting to our higher selves, we are able to restrain impulses, regulate desires, accept internal authority, and commune with our true, calm nature. By prioritizing this yogic state of mind, our relationship stresses diminish. Ultimately, staying true to our fundamental purpose saves us from the internal pain and suffering which inevitably affects our relationships.

Remember that each of us is in charge of our own thoughts and responses. Self-reliance is caring for the higher self first and taking 100 percent responsibility for ourselves. If a coworker is creating a disturbance within us, then it is *our own* disturbance. By accepting that simple fact, we are empowered to take action. When peace of mind is disrupted, we may choose a different state of mind and work toward it, such as returning to peace, contentment, or ease. Sometimes we need assistance; asking for answers or support is an aspect of self-reliance. Alternatively, we may take action to rectify a situation. This may involve discussing our concerns, offering directives for change, modifying the upsetting situation ourselves, or simply using it as a challenge to strengthen our internal virtues. Self-reliance means prioritizing the higher self, taking action on our own behalf, and asking for help as required.

Exercise: Self-Loving Yoga Postures

Practice this sequence during times of emotional unrest. Let go of any perfectionism or competition in your approach, which can lead to anxiety and limit deep, loving connections. Focus on the center of your chest and the corresponding place between your shoulder blades. Imagine yourself drawing comfort into those places, soothing and filling the chest and upper back then circulating to the rest of your body. Set aside any mental busyness until after practice. If your mind wanders, keep bringing it back to love. Allow the following yoga posture sequence to offer restfulness, joy of gentle movement, and a feeling of giving and receiving love.

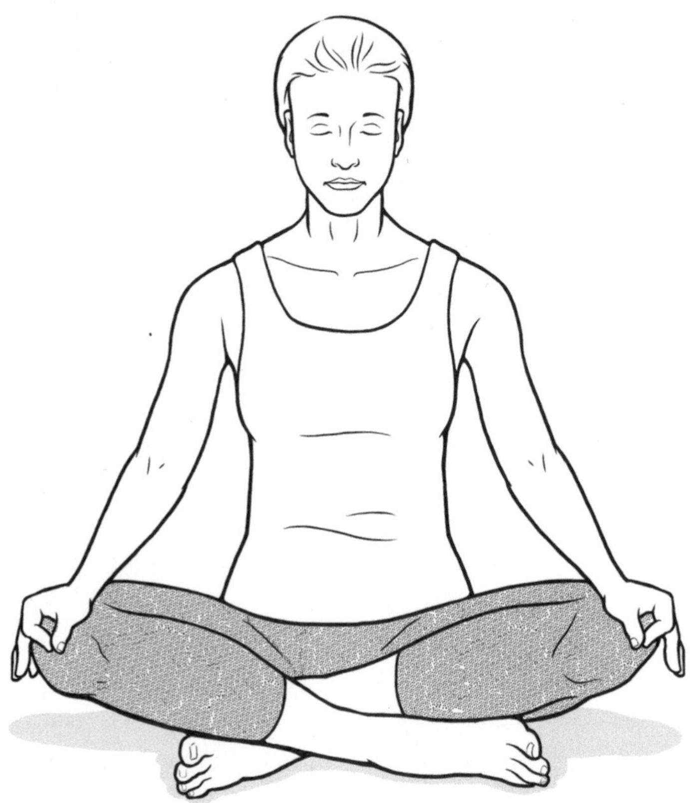

Figure 9.1
a. *Sukhasana* **(Easy Seated Pose)**

With a slight smile on your face and deep, rhythmic breathing, sit cross-legged with your hands resting comfortably on your knees. Take the time to reflect on what you are bringing with you to the mat: bodily sensations, quality of thoughts, emotional state, sense of connection and presence. Inhale deeply, focusing on drawing in goodness. Exhale fully, releasing all the obstacles to wellness. As your attention shifts to the depth and slowing rhythm of your breath, separate from thoughts and feelings in order to objectively witness them. Do this without judgment, without a need to change them.

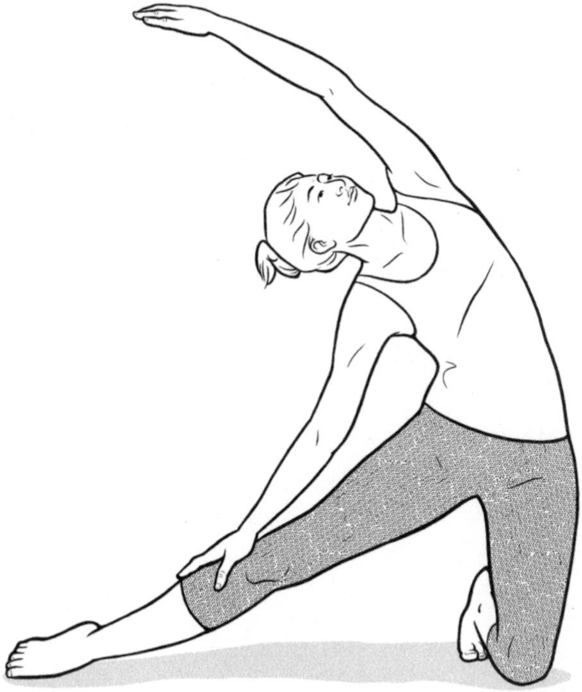

Figure 9.2
b. *Parighasana* (Gate Pose)

Stand on your knees, with a cushion or rolled mat beneath them for padding if needed. While the left hip remains directly above the left knee, extend one leg directly to the right side, maintaining alignment with the right hip, knee, and ankle. Slide the right hand down the extended leg and raise the left hand overhead. Without tilting forward or back, side bend over the extended leg. Inhale back to center and repeat the posture on the other side.

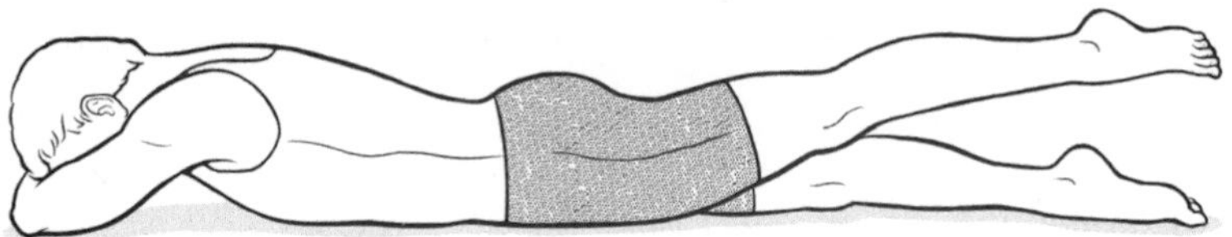

Figure 9.3
c. *Salabhsana* (Locust Pose), alternating legs

Rest on your abdomen, feet together or hip-width apart to protect your back. Your hands can make a pillow for your forehead or you can rest your palms down beside your hips. Inhale your right foot up, pointing your toes and keeping your knee straight and pointed toward the floor. Feel the strength in your mid-back extend out through the back of the leg and toes. Exhale your leg down with control, tucking in your chin. Repeat with your left leg. You can move slowly through this posture a few more times, breath by breath.

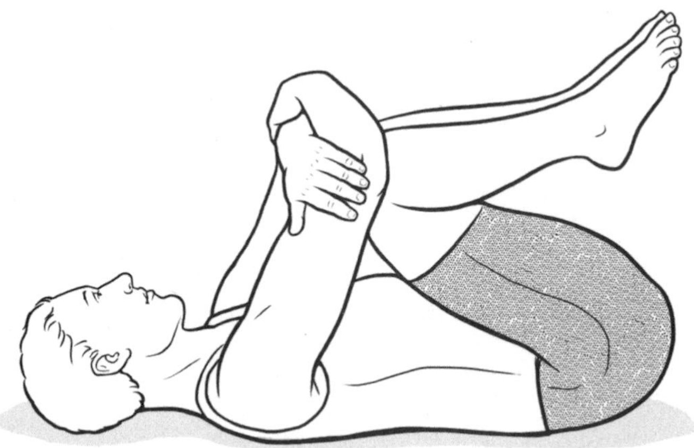

Figure 9.4
d. *Apanasana* (Knees-to-Chest Pose)

Roll onto your back. Bring both knees close to the chest with heels relaxed toward your seat and ankles side by side. Your arms may wrap around your shins or thighs to hug the legs a little closer. Rock gently from side to side to massage your back and soothe the emotions.

You may place your feet and arms on the ground and rock your knees slightly left and right while turning your face in the opposite direction.

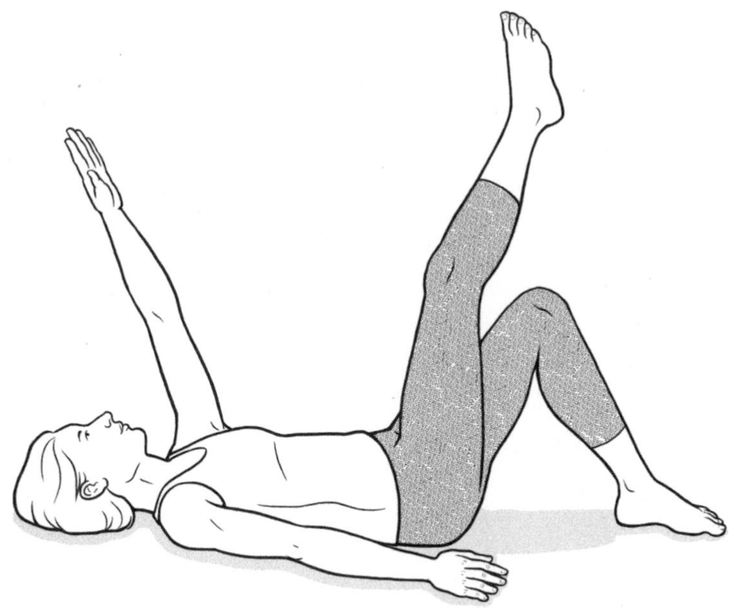

Figure 9.5
e. Inverted Action, raising opposite limbs

Remain on your back and float your right leg and left arm into the air, resting for a few breaths before trading sides. You may extend your left leg along the floor or keep the knee bent.

You may follow this practice with a letting-go relaxation, autosuggestion, or visualization to deepen the health benefits.

Remembering the Fundamental Purpose

Who is responsible for your health? You are! Of course, who else could it be? Keeping ourselves healthy is no small feat, as it involves a comprehensive approach to well-being, including accepting our limitations and illnesses. Numerous studies have demonstrated the link between emotional states, the nervous system, and immunity, or psychoneuroimmunology. Each system affects the others, enhancing and/or inhibiting processes elsewhere in the body. This type of science does not offer concrete plans of action such as medication or a specific action that will bring about a rapid healing. Instead, psychoneuroimmunology shows the importance of how the mind-body connection affects the immune system. The basic tenet is that a healthy range of emotions stimulates the immune system. However, if any emotion is repeated for longer than thirty minutes or is suppressed, a converse effect occurs on the immune system. Yoga helps us witness emotions without getting caught up in them, so we may honor our needs and maintain personal health.

Our primary adult relationship begins within our own minds. If we are not perfect at listening to others, it is unlikely that we are listening to our own thoughts and feelings. Self-talk is usually synonymous with self-criticism. We often hear "I am my own worst critic." Yoga's goal is to flip that around so that we can say, "I am my own best friend! I listen to my ideas, my feelings, and my dreams." We are always talking to ourselves, whether conscious of it or not. It is worth listening to what our thoughts are saying and cultivating uplifting internal messages. It is also important to listen deeply, tuning into the subtle messages of fatigue, hunger, enthusiasm, and affinity that may be expressed at any given moment. Ultimately, this deep listening hones our innate knowing and makes us better listeners to our loved ones.

Relationship to Loved Ones

For many people, especially kindhearted and empathetic folks, relationships bring on a great deal of stress. Wanting too much from our loved ones, even though it may be best for them, disconnects us from self-reliance in relationships because we are giving their choices the power to affect our internal climate. When we claim responsibility for our feelings we can manage them. By choosing to accept our loved ones unconditionally, connecting the purpose of our higher self to our relationships, we are less affected by our loved ones' behaviors and decisions. This gives us room to love them unconditionally. Our relationships with loved ones can be the greatest source of stress or a key aspect of our yoga practice. Allow your primary purpose and spiritual intention to nurture all of your relationships.

Exercise: Listen from the Heart

This exercise has the simplest instructions, but may be one of the hardest in the entire book. All you have to do is listen to someone else talk about their stress. Often, we jump in with advice or solutions; we love to help them find answers or make things better! Sometimes we get stressed by their stress, either because we are tired of hearing about it or because we don't want them to be hurt. The next time one of your loved ones complains or is upset or anxious, simply listen from your heart.

1. Follow these guidelines for listening:
    - Do not give advice. That puts more of a burden on you both.
    - Listen without a persona. Just hear what the other person is saying, without needing to come up with a response, joke, story, or validating comment.
    - Don't interrupt or relate their stress to yourself. Let this be their time to express. All you have to do is listen.
    - When your loved one is finished, you may ask a sincere question to explore the topic. "Have you tried...?" is advice and should be avoided. "Where do you think that's coming from?" is a sincere question.
2. You will get the most out of this exercise if you pay attention to the habits of your mind. Does it want to interrupt? Is it resonating with your loved one? Are you seeking solutions? Finding humor? Panicking? Simply notice, without needing to respond to your friend or your mind's habits.

Folks who relate to the yogic path of relationships and emotions are often "helpers," whether through career choice or simply by seeking opportunities to assist others. The desire to help turns into stress and anxiety when we are attached to outcomes. Unfortunately, kindhearted people tend to give too much assistance and promote dependence. Then we become depleted by continually giving to overly dependent people, which creates more stress for the loved ones we were trying to help in the first place. Our duty to loved ones does not involve depleting ourselves, as this violates our fundamental purpose.

We may feel uplifted by giving, which helps connect to our higher selves, but loved ones must be working toward their own wellness. The highest form of compassion is to help others help themselves so that they are not dependent on anyone. Give them space to foster their own fundamental purpose, then we can do the same for ours. This type of relationship empowers the people we love; they start to feel well and we help them develop their own spiritual connection and self-reliance. It is our duty to live spiritually, thereby inspiring the same in others. It is not our duty to create dependence or enable our loved ones, nor is it our duty to change them.

Tensions in loving relationships can be a main contributor to anxiety. It's okay to feel your feelings without being consumed by them. Truly allow your feelings to exist, get the message these emotions are sending you, and, without reacting to the feelings themselves, allow their message to guide you to the appropriate course of action. If someone is down or caught in a moment of selfishness, connect with them by recalling their goodness or kind actions they have taken in the past. You may not be able to do this at the same moment they are causing you stress; however, come back to compassion and peace as soon as possible. It is best to avoid negative thoughts about them, lest you become negative as well. Finding the virtue in others allows you to align with that virtue within and offers hope for the person you are facing.

Exercise: Heart Relaxation

This simple but powerful relaxation practice tunes you into your body, which can help take you away from being overly emotional. At the same time, it attunes you to your emotional center—your heart—and helps you feel relaxed there. This is a comforting practice when emotions are running high.

1. Settle into a relaxation posture and, once you are centered, begin to focus on the steady beating of your heart. If your mind wanders, simply bring it back to sensing your heartbeat.
2. As you become calm, notice your heart slowing. Even as you and your heart relax deeply, feel how it offers continual effort and support to keep you alive.
3. Relax into appreciation for and connection to your heart.

Loving with a Question

One of our yoga teachers has a teaching story about being in high school and having trouble dating. After facing some rejection, it dawned on this teenager that the situation may have to do with his behavior! He studied a book on relationships and learned to be kinder and more attentive to the needs of others. At the same time, his mother had been in psychotherapy and practiced what she learned in counseling on her teenage son. After school every day, she would have him express the ups and downs of things in long dialogues. He always felt better after these talks and her mini-therapy sessions made him appreciate the benefits of listening. As he began to practice listening to his dates and asking sincere questions, he realized that listening was the key. (The funny end of this story is that he had a lot of platonic girl friends!)

Listening creates intimacy and helps others feel affirmed, rather than breeding stress and anxiety through advice or a self-centered approach. You can be an extraordinary friend, lover, or coworker by taking the time to listen. Typically, the only people who really listen to you are those who really love you—and even that is rare! Some guidelines for listening are:

- Set a safe environment by asking questions before sharing your opinions. Your friend will trust you.

- When you do have an opinion about your friend's comment, ask more questions to test the validity of your opinion. Your interest in your friend's life will feel as though you care for him/her.
- Notice if you have formed your responses in your head before your friend is finished speaking. When you really listen to your friend's thoughts in the moment, s/he will feel honored and respected.
- Nurture a person's desires—or don't squash their thinking. This means that if someone says that they want you to help them, pause before agreeing or declining. Find out what the situation means to them. What are the details of the event? Learn about the deeper reason behind what they are asking. When you find out the root source of the person's wish, you will have helped them by listening even if you don't actually agree to the request.

Boundaries and Healing the Heart

Boundaries are key on the yogic path of relationships and emotions. They protect all concerned. When we know what we will and won't stand for, it becomes very simple to say no. Stay connected to your primary purpose as a fundamental internal boundary; this way, when you need to assert a boundary, you do so with the compassion and kindness of your higher self. Many people become upset when they have to draw a boundary or say no because we have been so conditioned to be "nice" and "helpful." We get stressed if we think we may not be doing something likeable. It is okay to feel this discomfort and at the same time uphold external boundaries through the four priorities (higher self, loved ones, work, community).

Internal boundaries may be harder to cultivate as they involve shifting perceptions, beliefs, and actions; however, your higher self, yoga friends, and commitment to the process will support you. When we have no boundaries, there is a sense of chaos and danger because there are no guidelines. Remember, boundaries are not mean—they help us all know where we stand, and this offers a true sense of security. Sometimes a firm, quiet "no, thank you" is the kindest thing we can offer ourselves and a relationship.

Exercise: Strengthening Interpersonal Boundaries

It can be very difficult for emotionally natured people to say no and set personal boundaries. The following exercise shifts your perspective on boundaries and helps you see that you may be more likeable and spiritual when you share the truth of your "no."

1. Think of a few people, living or dead, whether you have met them or not, whom you admire. What qualities do you admire about them? How are you like them? How were these admirable people's boundaries? Did others know where they stood?
2. Complete the following sentence: If I say no, I am afraid that ________________. An awareness of this fear allows you to address it. What's so scary about ______________ ? Most people are afraid of conflict, hurting others, or not being liked. As you grow to like yourself and become more confident in your reasons for boundaries, you will be less stressed by asserting them.
3. Sometimes it is hard to tell where our needs and issues end and another's begin. Just because someone is hurting doesn't mean we have to help. Someone else's problem is theirs, not ours. It is a kindly impulse to help, but it is impure if it causes self-harm. Say no to three people today. Notice how you handle it internally and externally. This boundary muscle takes some time to strengthen, but it is worth the practice.

What others think about you is none of your business. Most people are surprised the first time they hear this. "But they are thinking about *me*, of course it's my business. I need to set them straight. They need to know what a good person I am." From a self-reliance perspective, each of us is the master of our own feelings. Others can think and feel whatever they want about us; it's none of our business. What others believe about us is based on their own preconceived ideas, past experiences, likes and dislikes, desires, and expectations. How they perceive us is filtered through their own psychology and may have very little to do with objective reality.

When relationship issues arise, do not take it personally; rather, use it as an opportunity to practice objective neutrality, empathy, and self-reflection. Do not allow others' feelings or behavior toward you to cause pain or disconnection from the higher self you truly are. If there is truth in the other person's observations, you now have an impetus to act toward self-improvement. This is a gift! Ultimately, however, your role is to stay connected to your higher self and a sense of purpose and virtue in everyday life. You'll make mistakes, sometimes you'll fail, but there is no reason to be stressed as long as you continue to do your best.

Exercise: Self-Reliance in Relationships

Often we encounter people who unconsciously remind us of previous, or even current, relationships. Without realizing it, we may make assumptions about these people or ourselves in relation to them. Remember, we are the ones responsible for how we think and feel when relating to others throughout the day.

1. Think of a person you barely know whom you feel kindly toward. Does this person remind you of anyone?
2. Think of a difficult person in your life right now and journal your own beliefs and aversions.
3. Note how your preconceptions, past relationships, and beliefs create the problem within yourself.
4. Create a short statement to remind yourself to be self-reliant in keeping your inner environment neutral and not react to others.

5. Allow this affirming statement to become a meaningful part of your day, such as beginning or ending meditation, when taking a deep breath, during a relaxation before sleep, and especially when another person triggers you.

Relationship to the Divine

The higher self offers us great power. Contentment arises from uniting with the higher self so external relationships are easier to accept. Practice accepting small discomforts first, like rude people at the checkout counter, then shift that attitude of acceptance to larger difficulties, such as critical loved ones or a family member's addictive behavior. Even in dire situations, when we focus on an aspect of the higher self it clears our minds and elevates us away from the drama into intentional action. Rather than imposing our lower will onto something, we defer to the higher self, trusting in the divine order of the universe. In simpler terms, this is what we mean when we say go with the flow. Although this may not heal a loved one's illness or make a curmudgeonly person friendly, it does offer us the calm of knowing that we can only control ourselves, thereby choosing a state of peace or compassion. Being self-reliant enough to align with our higher nature makes all relationships divine.

Even the best-intentioned person will make mistakes that hurt others. There will always be pain in this life; it is the nature of earthly existence and there is no sense being stressed by it. Yoga philosophy reminds us to make the distinction between the earthly realm and the divine so that we are not so anxious about material problems. There is a difference between pain, which is inevitable, and suffering, which is a choice. When we suffer, we lose connection to the higher self and the virtue in all situations—this is scary. When we connect our awareness to a spiritual principle, there is just a pure feeling of pain and then a clear decision on how to adapt to the new situation. Nothing to be afraid of! This constant awareness of the divine in all situations is the most difficult feat for a human being to achieve. Our own constant internal vigilance and self-study are required to overcome the tendency to suffer or fear future hurt.

Self-reliance is key in dealing with difficult people. If they seem difficult, it is because we have become difficult. Remember, nothing external, including grumpy coworkers, aggressive drivers, or judgmental in-laws, has the power to upset our peace of mind unless we give it that power. We maintain our power by being self-reliant in regarding the higher truth of a situation, guided by compassion and acceptance. For example, if you work with a grumpy critic and let them be grumpy, there is no stress in responding to them. There is no inference into why they are critical around you or intent behind it. You don't need to control the grumpiness or protect yourself from criticism because these things arise in the other person. Your role is to stay connected to your higher self, be nurtured by spirit, and allow that fullness to shine through you.

A key to accepting difficult others is to look at any situation from the other person's point of view. Within each of us is the firm belief that what we are doing is right. It is unwise for us to make snap judgments about others' actions; the external behavior is only a tiny piece of what is actually going on within a person. What we often find is that the biggest bully is the one with the deepest pain and insecurity. Be active and ask the other person questions to find out their perspective. Perhaps there is a personal tragedy. Maybe the person is self-centered and unaware of their harmful impact on others and needs to be confronted. Simply listen and do not advise or interpret. It is not possible to accept anyone whom you do not understand. Once a situation is clear, acceptance is easier and difficult people stop being difficult because your perceptions have changed.

Pay attention to your thoughts, reactions, and preferences in order to understand the events, people, and time of day that disconnect you from your higher self. Also understand the simple practices that are reconnecting, such a deep breath, affirmation, focus on a virtue, and prayer. By getting to know ourselves in this way, we are less swayed by the habit of anxious responses.

We now have the tools for recognizing when we are engaging in thoughts and behaviors that do not relate to the higher self. To avoid becoming overwhelmed, choose one simple intention to practice. Remember that countering deep-seated tendencies toward stress and anxiety requires regular and diligent practice because the subconscious mind operates according to suggestions that have been programmed from early childhood, even when they are harmful and cause suffering. Do not indulge or rationalize negative influences, but rather, cultivate the opposite. On the other hand, sometimes it is necessary to feel a negative emotion. In surrendering to the emotion, you allow a deeper level of understanding to surface. (If this does not occur in time, you may choose to consult with a counselor.) Ask, "What is anxiety trying to tell me to change? How might stressful situations help me learn to take better care of myself?" Even if you can't change things, you can use the opportunity to practice equanimity and nonattachment to negative reactions. An emotion can be acknowledged without giving it control. It's not that yogis don't have emotions, but that they understand their emotions very well. Becoming aware of our emotions affects how we respond to circumstances in life.

There is a famous story of a distressed disciple. The sage threw a handful of salt into a glass of water and told the disciple to drink. The water tasted very bitter. The sage threw another handful of salt, this time into the ocean, and told the disciple to drink that. Although it was still salty, the ocean water did not have the same intense bitterness. This is likened to us, either handling problems on our own, like that limited glass of water handling the salt, versus remembering that we are a part of a huge ocean of life and that vast allegiance takes away the bitterness. It is an analogy for relying on the higher self.

Self-reliance helps us tolerate pain by strengthening us on all levels. Taking responsibility and connecting to the higher self helps us rise above our human nature and protects us from the impulse to stress about life. This requires willpower and the cultivation of positive thoughts and actions, resulting in a sense of confidence and competence rather than stress and anxiety. Self-reliance comes with a humble feeling of achievement, satisfaction, and wisdom, enabling us to face pain in relationships and transform it into personal strength.

The following activities are recommended for those of an emotional nature. These, and many other heart-centered activities, help harness the emotions and connect to divine love.

- Laugh!
- Engage in devotional singing or chanting where folks free themselves to express.
- Rhythm and music are powerful, whether you are playing or listening.
- Spend time in nature and be in awe of its beauty, geometry, biology, and intricacy.
- Practice Hatha Yoga.
- Meditate or focus on breathing deeply.
- Recall deeply religious and peak experiences. Utilize your deep beliefs to motivate daily practices and uplift your mind.
- Create! Color with crayons, fingerpaint, or take painting lessons.
- Explore other ways that you reconnect to your higher self and realign your emotions and spirit.

Breathe, Then *Respond*

Highly emotional people have a reputation for being too sensitive and expressive in relationships. This can look like over-talking, crying, or rage-filled outbursts. A simple trick to avoid being judged as an overly emotional person in relationships is to take a breath before responding. Even if someone has asked a question, you have the right to reflect before answering. This is a more subtle aspect of listening from the heart, where you have the chance to truly listen to yourself. Typically, a single breath before responding can remove most of the charge from an otherwise automatic—and usually over-dramatic—reaction. When we understand the need underlying the stress, we are able to feed ourselves the corresponding virtue, which inevitably shines through our response. Ultimately, emotions are simply one stream of information that can lead us to connection with the higher self.

Exercise: Shifting Stress

We all wish to avoid stress. This is biologically built into us! However, there is a difference between a true life-threatening stress and the emotion of stress that can be triggered by any number of life events. This exercise is a chance for you to scrutinize stressful patterns in life. By understanding the common thread, you are better able to respond with clarity the next time you are stressed.

1. Select a stressor that you have an aversion to. Allow yourself to truly feel that dislike, observing it like an anthropologist in order to understand. Remember that by feeling the pain, we are able to understand it. You may journal these feelings.
2. Remember a stressor from six months ago that you felt aversion to and repeat the emotional observation process, possibly journaling feelings.
3. Recall a stressor from your teen years that created an aversion, feel it, and journal the feelings.
4. As you review your perceptions or journal entries notice the similarities and differences of these feelings. What do the similarities teach you about yourself, your stress, and your aversions? Note that the historical similarities you just discovered may relate to a past unmet need.
5. What virtue or spiritual feeling soothes that pattern of stress and aversion? From now on when that feeling arises, let it be your friend, reminding you to call upon your higher self and an uplifted feeling or virtue.

Harness Your Emotional Power

It's funny, but the nervous system can't tell the difference between excitement and anxiety. Think about it: your heart starts pounding, breath speeds up, pupils dilate, adrenaline gets pumping… are you having a panic attack or going to see your favorite musician? The story we tell ourselves can be the difference between stress and passion. All situations are subject to interpretation and our habitual thought patterns tend to color all of our experiences. For example, if you think you are an anxious person, then the flush of getting a promotion winds up attributed to it being a fearful, rather than celebratory, experience. Challenge yourself to call anxiety "enthusiasm."

In order to harness the power of your emotions, become aware of the things you fear, even at the most subtle level. At first, you may notice how anxiety takes you away from your yoga practice by motivating escapism and unhealthy behaviors. Do not dwell on these anxieties; rather, step back and see the bigger picture of life. What information is contained in these emotions? What action is it offering in order to improve your life and connect to the higher self? Accept all feelings and learn from this ongoing awareness rather than succumbing to stress. When we use the information from our emotions, we employ their power to create positive change in our lives.

Another way to harness and use our emotional power is through joy. Laughter is highly therapeutic. It boosts cardiovascular health and circulation, decreases residual tension, amplifies immune function by reducing cortisol and increasing the flow of lymph, and improves mood with a natural endorphin release. The many benefits of reducing cortisol and increasing endorphins are well-documented. Suffice it to say, it keeps you happy, confident, healthy, and resilient to stress.

Laughter yoga can be practiced anytime, by anyone. It helps to begin with a grin, to get you into a happier mood. Bouncing on the toes and raising the arms overhead also help the laughter come more easily. You may perform a typical sequence of yoga postures, noticing the level of flexibility and relaxation the laughter brings!

We recommend you try a formal laughter yoga class. Laughter yoga teachers are well-trained with humor and techniques to keep you giggling the entire class. We walk away from laughter yoga connected to joy, well-being, and the higher self.

Exercise: Life's Great Comedy

Many families use humor to diffuse tension: whenever folks become too stressed out or angry, you can rest assured someone will break into a comedy bit. Impressions, jokes, humorous observations, and repeating funny lines from heartening movies are all techniques we can use to make each other laugh throughout the day. Use the following questions to help connect you to your own sense of humor and find more laughter each day.

1. What are your top five favorite comedies? Which comedy characters are you most like? Why? What makes you laugh? Is it improvisation, irony, slapstick, surrealism, observational comedy, snappy dialogue?
2. Consider how your anxiety or other uncomfortable emotions also have a funny side. Look for opportunities throughout the day to turn passing stresses into jokes. Chuckle at the ineffective coping strategies you observe in yourself. You may exaggerate the potential bad outcomes of the situation. Are you being blind to positive alternatives? Tease yourself into a higher perspective on things.

Like-Minded Support

How do you spend your free time? When you are hanging out with friends, what do you do together? Do these activities uplift you? How are activities different from one group of friends to the other? What about the times of day when you do the activities? How do they keep you connected to your higher self? More time in uplifting activities limits stress in life and cultivates a healthy relationship with others and the higher self. Connect with your friends when they are most virtuous and nurture your relationships as you make spiritual choices. This encourages them too!

In situations such as work or family gatherings, you may seek out like-minded people and join with them. A schoolteacher from our yoga community began to avoid the staffroom, where many other teachers would complain about the work and the children. This yoga practitioner gathered with a small group of teachers who also found the environment in the staffroom grating and stressful. This handful of teachers began taking their lunches in the library, supporting each other where necessary, brainstorming about ways to contribute to the school, and sharing small victories that were occurring in the classroom. They remained friendly with all the other teachers, but appreciated their uplifting staff area.

As we make yoga a bigger part of our lives, it is beneficial to have yoga friends as well. These people speak the same language and understand the subtle but powerful effects yoga has on our lives. Yoga friends encourage us to stay connected to our higher selves and share a bond of joy.

Exercise: Community

Community is essential on the path of personal growth. We all need like-minded people to share ideas, trials, and victories with. Contemplate who in your world can join you on this path out of anxiety and into greater alignment with the higher self.

1. It is important to seek out others who are also on a path of self-realization. Whom do you know who is also working on becoming a more balanced person? Think of friends and relatives, coworkers, and also friends of friends or people you have lost contact with over the years.
2. Continue to make small steps in the direction of avoiding people who indulge in gossip, complaining, or worry, and instead connecting to emotionally uplifted people.
3. Who on the outskirts of your life seems like a balanced, authentic person? What small action could you take to connect with this person? Saying hello in the hall, commenting on the weather, sending a quick email, or sitting with them at lunch are simple ways of building rapport.

As you continue to free yourself from stress and anxiety, you will grow stronger in your relationships with others. Continue to use the exercises in this chapter to stay relaxed and conscious. Stay connected to your intention, speak your truth, listen deeply, and remember to reach out to your higher self and the Divine. Aligning with your inner truth will improve your relationships and support you in reaching out to the community at large, to both offer and receive support.

Chapter Summary

1. Relationships are a major source of stress.
2. Stress can create issues in the body. Emotions and health are linked: a somatic reality.
3. External situations need not dictate our internal emotional state.
4. Caring for our own higher self is the first step in caring for others.
5. Take 100 percent responsibility for your emotions and actions.
6. Yoga postures remind us how to nurture and love ourselves.
7. Truly loving others means cultivating a feeling of love, not stress. Listening to difficult people also enhances compassion and smoothes out our reactions to relationships.
8. Listening to our inner selves, accepting our emotions, and staying healthy gives us strength to be loving and helpful to those around us.
9. Relax with self-love by listening to your own slow, constant heartbeat.
10. Filter pain and discomfort through the Divine. Practice sitting with uncomfortable emotions while keeping your spirituality in mind. There are many personally meaningful ways of connecting to the Divine.
11. Healthy boundaries demonstrate love to ourselves and others. Boundaries protect everyone.

12. No longer assume that you are an anxious person. Anger, excitement, and enthusiasm can feel the same on a physiological level.
13. Others' thoughts about us are none of our business. We are subject to others' projections and vice versa. If you feel an aversion to someone, be self-reliant and examine your own history.
14. Hold a spiritual intention for relationships. Allow this higher emotion to color all of your interactions with ease and love.
15. Emotions are a terrific source of information and guidance when attended to with a calm, open mind.
16. Laughter and humor channel the emotions in profoundly healing ways.
17. Relationships with like-minded people support our spiritual development and help ease our emotional stresses.

Now that you have studied your anxiety in relation to the five yogic paths (psychology, intellect, health, work, and relationships/emotions), we will look at practical ways you can keep this yoga therapy lifestyle vital. The more we live in alignment, the better our lives get, for as long as we live!

Part III: Making Yoga Therapy a Lifestyle

So far, this book has given you yoga philosophy, personal insight, and practical techniques to free yourself from stress and anxiety. Part III supports you in carrying these strategies through your life so that stress and anxiety do not return. Chapter 10 identifies common barriers to progress, and Chapter 11 helps you solidify your vision of a peaceful future! Complete the exercises and enquiries from this section as an affirmation of all the work you have done as well as your potential for a life free from stress and anxiety.

Chapter 10

Overcoming Barriers to the Anxiety-Free Life

Rich with exercises, this chapter works with you to address the common barriers to progress. The main thing standing between you and a stress-free life is you! Now that you have an understanding of how yoga therapy removes stress and anxiety, your role is to continue the process to freedom. We capitalize on what you have learned throughout this book in order to gain the utmost benefit for your anxiety-free life. Complete the exercises of this chapter and support yourself in removing the main obstacles we tend to put in our own way!

Know Your Own Mind's Tricks

Did anyone ever tell you "You can't teach an old dog new tricks"? Puppies are malleable and they're continually learning about their environment. They create new habits every day. It's probably right that teaching a puppy another new thing is easy but teaching the older dog is harder once its habits are ingrained.

Patterns are ingrained right down into our physiology. Quite literally, the brain and nervous system have patterns embedded in them. We can't always change our internal or external patterns immediately. However, we can change our reaction to the pattern. Think about it this way: when something in life happens, you react to it, usually in the same way you reacted to it the last time it happened and the hundred similar times before that. For example, when you have too much to do and someone asks you for one more thing, your habit may be to feel stress of some kind, then react to that stress with well-rehearsed behaviors such as anger, eating, smoking, crying, or any range of responses. Even though there are many responses available, chances are you return to the same few choices continually. Stress and anxiety become a patterned answer to a situation.

If instead you remember to greet that stress with acceptance, your brain feels acceptance rather than stress. A new pathway begins to develop in your brain, one of acceptance rather than stress or anxiety. When you do the exercises in this book, the likelihood is you will get really anxious from trying to get rid of your anxiety because that pattern is there. When you bring a level of self-acceptance to the process, it will cause you to be patient. You won't expect an immediate change and the stress is easier to cope with. Create new behaviors from your higher, patient self. However you react to a situation is simply the initial thought. Any range of human emotions is acceptable! From that initial thought, let the higher self discern the emotions and guide you to a more peaceful place.

Exercise: Mind Tricks

The more we understand the habits underlying our anxiety, the easier it is to be neutral toward the internal chatter. Our perceptions of situations are imperfect, based on our past experiences, likes, dislikes, desires, and expectations. In this way, the mind plays tricks on us, preventing us from viewing a neutral reality where we have more response options than simply stress. In this exercise, experiment with your mental habits and understand the tricks your mind might be playing on you.

1. Recall a time when you misunderstood another person or a situation. Journal the emotions you were feeling at the beginning of the misunderstanding.

2. As the situation progressed and the other person tried to clarify or you realized the situation may not be what it originally seemed, how did your feelings change? There are many ways you may have reacted; do your best to recall the truth and record it for learning.
3. Journal any insights about the roots of your own automatic reactions. Were you raised to believe or react that way? Were you hurt in the past and are overly sensitive now? Do you fit separate situations into a single world view or personal story? Each of us has a biased mind and we do not even record most objective information accurately; it passes through our personal filters first. As we witness this phenomenon, we are less subject to the mind's programmed reactions.
4. When you notice yourself telling a story about a situation—don't believe the mind's tricks! Rather, witness the thoughts and feelings that are present. Receive their message and continue cultivating an objective, relaxed perspective.

Resistance to Healing

Resistance is a part of the healing process. For whatever reason, even when we see that our practices are making us better, we sometimes avoid healthy behaviors and attitudes. As you have likely experienced in your own practice, exploring uncomfortable emotions is not always easy. It can be painful and scary. That is why so many of us, even longtime yoga practitioners, do our best to avoid our wounds.

Cameron, a dedicated yoga teacher, turned to research whenever emotions got too uncomfortable. When dealing with a sick parent, stress mounted quickly. Instead of unwinding this anxiety and working through the many feelings that were arising, Cameron turned to the Internet for information on the symptoms and prognosis of the parent's illness, how to cope, what the treatment options were, and so on. While on the computer, Cameron would also play games, visit social media sites, and answer work emails instead of eating and going to bed. As this habit of turning to the Internet whenever feelings arose became ingrained, Cameron became more tired during the day, less grounded, and highly irritable. For a time, emotions became so uncomfortable that the pattern of turning to the Internet started to cause problems in the marriage, with the children, and even at work. Cameron soon realized that resistance to feeling the pain was actually creating more pain and began setting aside time to journal, relax, talk to friends, and practice yoga poses to remove stress. By cultivating those healthier coping strategies, Cameron was a stronger support to the sick parent, a better spouse, parent, and employee, and most importantly, more aligned with the higher self. Although there was pain in life, Cameron was able to move through it with grace and determination, rather than stress and avoidance.

Exercise: Getting to the Root of Resistances

It is ironic that our avoidance of feelings, or resistance, actually causes much of the pain and stress! When we are able to greet our emotions as teachers, resistance falls away and new understandings can be formed. This practice of moving through resistance helps us to accept life as it is. The following exercise helps you understand the source of your resistances and offers a template for transcending them.

1. Select a situation that you do not accept. There may be many; just pick one. Journal your habitual beliefs and frustrations with it. Be honest, no matter what comes to mind. You may notice thoughts that you don't truly believe. If they are in you somewhere, they are worth examining.
2. Notice the emotions that arise with the thoughts. Stay with these feelings even though they are uncomfortable. Breathe deeply to connect with your higher self and witness the feelings. Name the emotions in your journal and acknowledge what happens in your body as you feel them. Are the feelings associated with likes/dislikes, expectations, or desires? Do they remind you of other biases you possess?

3. Reflecting more deeply on these feelings now, when is the first time you remember feeling this way? In other words, how are these emotions familiar to you? What specific past experiences relate to these emotions? Stay with this exercise even though it is uncomfortable—remember that emotions are simply information; even though they are uncomfortable, they cannot harm you.
4. From this reflection, can you see what you really want? What is the deeper desire that is coming through you? Now imagine yourself moving in the direction of that deep internal calling. Begin to color it with a desire for acceptance. Feel yourself wanting to accept yourself and your life. Notice that acceptance, and the peace of mind and control it brings, actually fits into your authentic desire. The resistance and pain do not fit the desire; rather, those feelings and behaviors were messengers so you could discover what was really going on. Now difficult situations are transformed into learning opportunities!

Exercise: Hearing What Your Mind is Trying to Say

There is a paradox where feeling anxious can be a key to ridding ourselves of anxiety. Anxious feelings, worry, fear, and the like are healthy messages from the emotional world. They tell us that something is amiss and requires adjustment. Because of our fast-paced, disconnected lifestyle, we might never look at how to balance ourselves were it not for stress ringing the alarm bell. The information our emotions offer can guide us on the path of removing stress. Our feelings give ongoing feedback about the direction we are going. The following exercise gives you the steps to use your emotions as tools for stress removal.

1. Every emotion offers information and direction. We must be sensitive enough to discern what we are truly feeling to glean

the information from the emotion. Select an emotion from the previous exercise or any strong feeling you are currently experiencing. Take a few deep breaths to observe the emotion, where it is in your body, its intensity, and so on.

2. What is the emotion telling you about your life? Journal freely for up to 20 minutes, without letting the pen stop. Trust the emotions to give you deep insight about how to free yourself from your current situation and move into acceptance. Hint: When your pen pauses, you are about to have a breakthrough. Instead of stopping, write *anything* and soon enough, an insight will arise.

Exercise: What You Are Already Doing!

Have you ever thought of what you would do if you won the lottery? Or how things might be if you had a new home, job, or relationship? As you read this book, are you thinking about what your life will be like once you integrate these lessons and lifestyle shifts? Thoughts about the future can be a big distraction during the process of removing stress. The temptation to daydream looms over each day as we wish things were different already! Once the train of future thoughts begins, it can derail your progress in removing stress and anxiety from your life. To help with this process of accepting and staying present with current reality, do the exercise below. When you secure your direction, a deeper acceptance arises, knowing you are moving toward freedom.

1. Chances are that you, like most of us, give more weight to your mistakes than to your sound actions. This skewed perspective is demoralizing and undermines all the effort you have put into creating your healthy lifestyle. Right now, list your healthy habits.

2. Affirm these rewarding behaviors by congratulating yourself, reciting affirmations, smiling, or praying. Let this uplifted feeling, based on the efforts you make, strengthen your existing discipline.
3. Smile right now, a huge grin, and notice the difference it makes to your sense of well-being. Remember that we all do some healthful activities, but it is impossible to do everything perfectly all the time. Feeling inadequate is counterproductive, while basking in the joy of what you do makes room for more of the same!
4. Build from this strong foundation. Slowly experiment with new behaviors by introducing them one at a time. When the new behavior becomes a routine, you are ready to add another. This is a gradual, permanent process of uplifting your lifestyle. Remain positive as you appreciate all the good things you do practice—it matters!

Any successful athlete or musician will tell you that visualization is central to their excellent performance. Envisioning our actions beforehand trains the brain to execute the plan in reality. Amazingly enough, performing an action or simply visualizing it tends to activate almost the same areas of the brain. Even more amazing is the fact that *watching* someone perform an action activates similar areas of the brain in both the observer and the person doing it. Maybe that is why we feel calm when we watch someone meditate and stressed when we see others who are stressed.

Worry and stress are ways of rehearsing future pain. It is possible to take that habit of fretting and transform it into a tool for an anxiety-free life. By visualizing your life without anxiety, you are mentally rehearsing new, relaxed responses to stressors before they even arise. Later, in times of stress, the mental habit of being calm in the face of stress comes to the fore.

❀ Exercise: Image of an Anxiety-Free Life

Inspiration comes from knowing where we are headed. By imagining the details of a life without anxiety, you are able to take clear action in that direction. For the following exercise, allow yourself to be as creative and elaborative as possible.

1. Draw or describe in a journal, with as many details as possible, the details of your everyday life, free from anxiety. You may include ideas about new responses to current anxiety triggers as well as general attitudes. What is on your mind when you wake up? What do you see in the mirror? What do others notice about you? How do you respond to irritations or difficulties throughout the day? What is your general sense of connection to your higher self?
2. Review this image of your anxiety-free life regularly, especially in times when you are losing motivation or feeling resistant to the efforts required to remove stress from your life.

❀ Exercise: Leveraging

The word "leverage" means "to use something to its highest advantage." This exercise maximizes the energy of your current lifestyle, which likely has aspects that are useful in managing your stress levels and bouts of anxiety, to carve a path away from stress.

1. What is already working for you? Write a list of these things and post or carry it somewhere accessible, in case stress mounts. Simple reminders are beneficial in times when we are unsure how to proceed with a balanced state of mind.
2. The past may also offer clues to how you can remove stress. Think of a time in your life when you rarely felt anxious, or felt like you had it under better control. What was different about your daily habits at that time? Who was around you? What were you interested in? How did you spend your free

time? By retracing the steps of what you did when healthy, you are readily able to reintroduce those past healthful habits.

Returning to an old habit, no matter how long it's been since you had it, is much easier than creating new habits where there is no foundation at all in the brain. There might be many reasons why returning to the familiar is easier than developing something new. One reason is that we can visualize a place we have been before. When we think of this calm, healthy place we are also visualizing the people around us and we might even imagine smells and sounds. This awakens feelings of pleasure and activation of the parasympathetic nervous system. This can be an immediate response and connects or activates certain areas of the brain in a certain pattern—areas that have been connected before. No matter how long ago it was, the brain can still find the connections. To build new neural pathways and connections takes much more deliberate practice. While we know from the recent science of neuroplasticity that the brain can develop new pathways in a fairly short time, it still takes longer to develop these pathways and make them easily available than it does to reawaken old pathways triggered by pleasant experiences. It's easier to recreate what once was than to develop something completely novel.

Life Balance

Anxiety and stress are evidence of a life out of balance. The issue may not relate to external balance, but rather, an internally balanced perspective on life. It is natural for demands, schedules, and emotional equilibrium to shift on a continual basis. When we accept this, we meet life with a more balanced perspective and less stress, no matter what is happening externally.

Remember, you have control of your emotional reactions to situations and your anxiety may be regulated by your reactions, be they calm or stressed. Strive to minimize charged situations that steal your sense of calm. Be sure to take time to enjoy positive emotions with laughter, fun, and free time—even if it feels lazy! Creating time for ourselves is key in understanding what we truly need for a balanced life.

Yoga Home Practice

A basic home practice is one of the most impactful things you can do to maintain your peace of mind and confidence in everyday life. Home practice need not be a prolonged business—ten to fifteen minutes is often enough. Begin paying attention to your day and seeing where you can slot in that brief period of time. Would first thing in the morning fit? Right after work? Or is a bedtime practice best for you?

Once you have determined a time to practice, find a place. Don't get too hung up on creating an ideal location right now (although have fun with it if it inspires you!). Whether it's at the foot of the bed, beside an armchair, in the basement, or halfway under the piano, it doesn't matter! Just find a place.

Now that you have a time and a place, begin spending a brief period every day going through poses, focusing on your breath, doing a meditation, reflecting, paying attention to what awakens in you and what emotions and feelings surface, journaling, or taking in some spiritual reading. Some days your practice may be sipping tea and looking out the window, and other days it might be going for a walk. What is most important is that you take time all to yourself for quietude and self-observation. Notice the effect this has on slowing down life and inoculating you against pressure and emotional pain.

If you have only ever attended yoga classes, the sequencing and specifics of yoga postures might be very confusing. Some students love yoga so much they spend ten minutes in the car after class writing down what they can remember about the sequences, which never wind up being complete. We recommend you spend a good deal of time at a bookstore selecting a yoga posture book that inspires you.

The basics of a yoga posture practice are simple:

1. Keep your brain-breath-body connection vital. Remain aware.
2. Warm up your spine in all five directions (upward, forward, backward, lateral, and twist).

3. Sequence counterpostures. For example, follow forward bends with backward bends, and what you do to the left side, repeat on the right.
4. Relax at the end, to assimilate benefits.

Relaxation is a key component in integrating the benefits of yoga practice. Similarly, we must receive adequate rest in life in order to stay healthy, assimilate our experiences, and release stress and anxiety.

Exercise: Proper Rest

Fatigue may interfere with your commitment to home practice. When we are very tired, we don't want to spend our free time doing "one more thing," even if that thing is deeply enjoyable and beneficial. We are a sleep-deprived culture. Electricity is probably the main reason for this problem, but long working hours, not enough recreation, and facing high levels of stress from the moment we awaken all contribute to our reluctance to go to bed on time. Furthermore, many people are unable to sleep deeply enough or properly enough. Accepting that you may be sleep-deprived is the first step in removing this barrier to home practice.

1. Make your bedroom as dark as possible. To help your glands function optimally and to restore your body, ensure that when you open your eyes at night, you only see black. You can install blackout shades or even cut cardboard to the size of your windows. Get rid of the glowing alarm clock.
2. If you fall asleep during yoga relaxations, your body needs the rest. It's okay to fall asleep (just set a timer at home if you have to be anywhere afterward!). Receive the rest in the moment it's happening and use it as a signal to evaluate your resting habits. Can you go to bed earlier? Is it best to reduce the number of activities in your schedule? When can you fit a fifteen-minute nap into your average day?

3. During rest, we assimilate experiences, unravel emotions, and consolidate learning. Without proper rest, we tax the emotions and nervous system, inevitably clouding the intellect and wearing down the body. What is one small shift you can make today to create more rest in your life?

Exercise: Yoga Posture Routine for Bedtime

Certain yoga postures are designed to downregulate the nervous system so the body can rest and heal. For folks who have no other time in the day for a yoga posture home practice, a bedtime routine is an efficient way to incorporate yoga into everyday life. It sets the body into "rest and digest" mode and soothes the mind. This prepares us for a deeper, higher quality sleep as we release the stress of the day rather than carrying it into our dreams.

Follow this sequence to help you retire in a more relaxed state. As you become accustomed to these movements and understand a wider range of yoga postures, you may adapt it to suit your needs. Place your mat, if you have one, directly beside your bed so that you may slip right under the covers for relaxation and drift off to sleep. (Bonus: The next morning when you rise, your mat is right there for you to do a handful of gentle waking-up movements.)

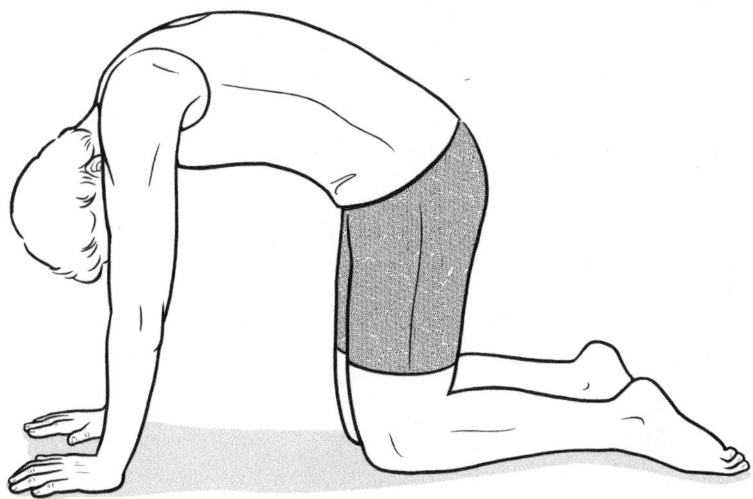

Figure 10.1a
Marjariasana **(Cat Pose)**

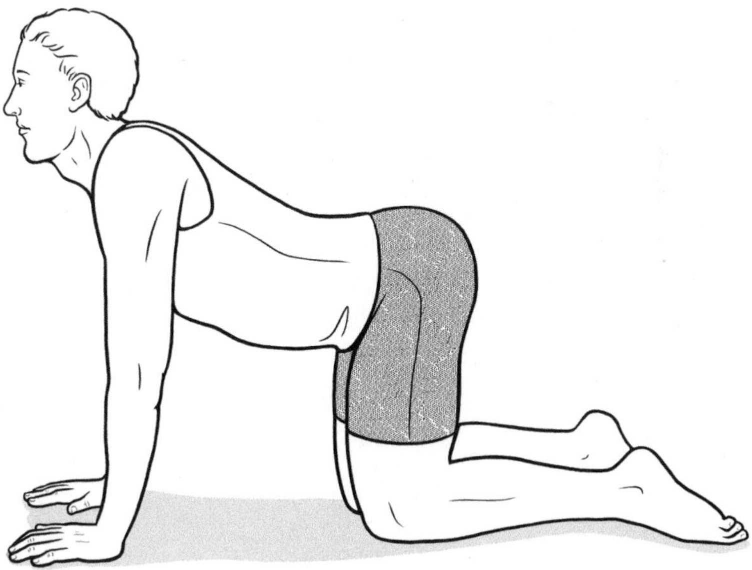

Figure 10.1b
Bitilasana **(Cow Pose)**

Begin on all fours, hands under shoulders with fingers spread wide and knees under hips. Exhale and round your back upward, tucking pelvis and chin inward as your navel pulls up. Inhale and reverse the arch in your back, tilting the tailbone up and reaching the chin forward, then upward. Connect the movement to breath as you continue. The deeper the breath, the slower the movement, and the more calming this will be.

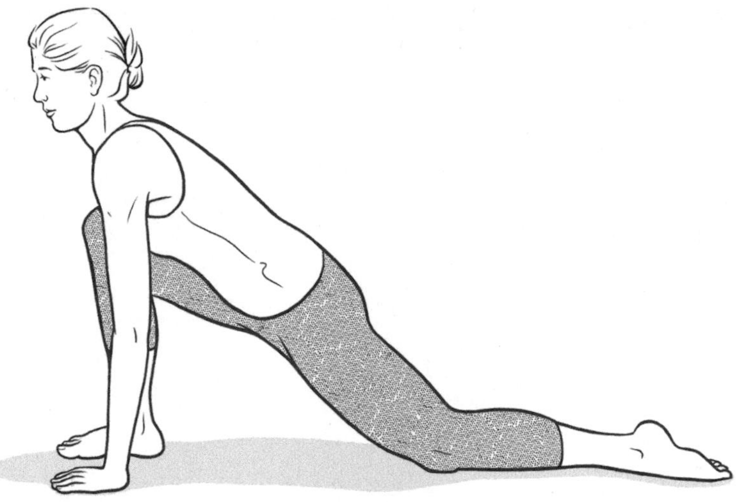

Figure 10.2a
2. *Anjaneyasana* (Low Lunge with side bend variation)

From the all-fours position, bring your right foot into the space between your hands. The knee is over the ankle and your front foot is flat on the floor. Your left leg extends back to rest the knee and the top of the foot on the floor. Look forward or rest your neck down. Once steady, lift your torso by walking your hands to the front thigh or raising your arms overhead. Gently begin to ease your torso to the right. If steady, you can raise your left arm alongside your head. Come out of the side bend, place your hands back on the floor, and trade sides.

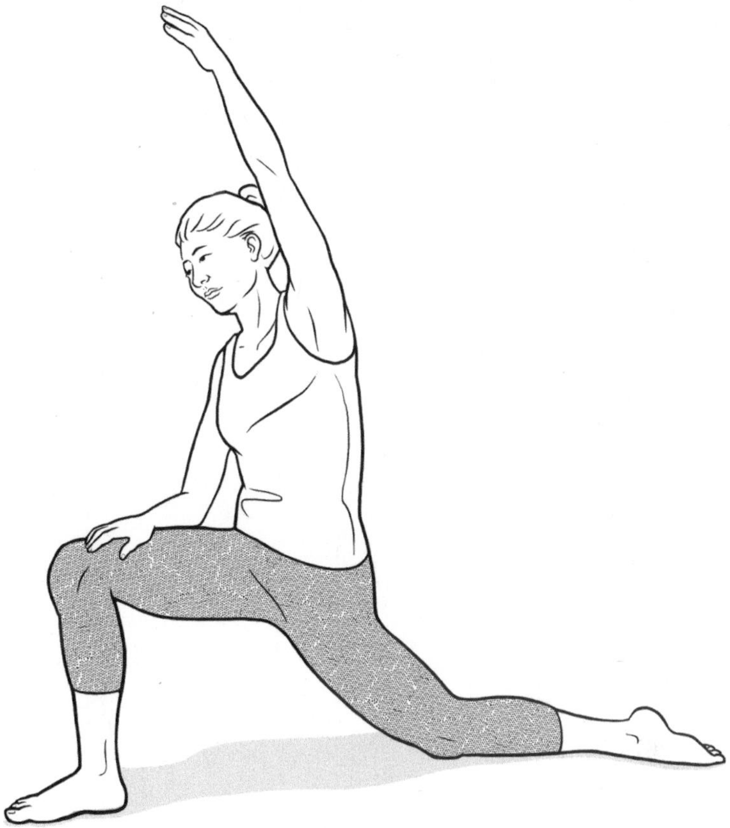

Figure 10.2b
2. *Anjaneyasana* (Low Lunge with side bend variation)

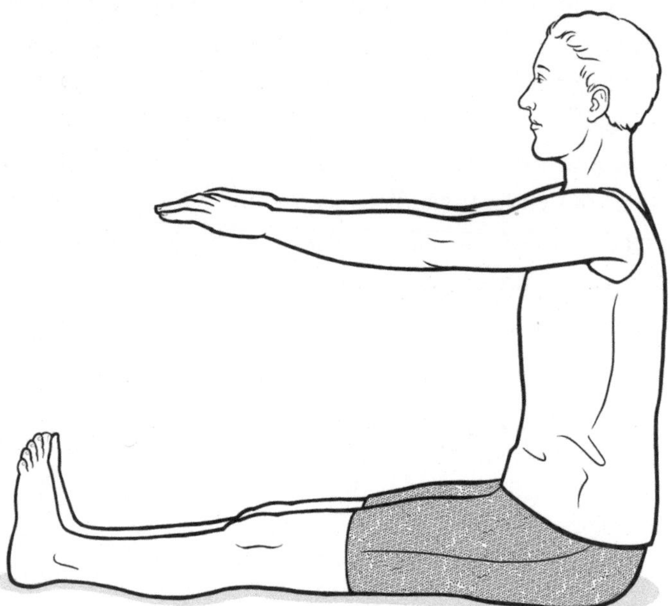

Figure 10.3a

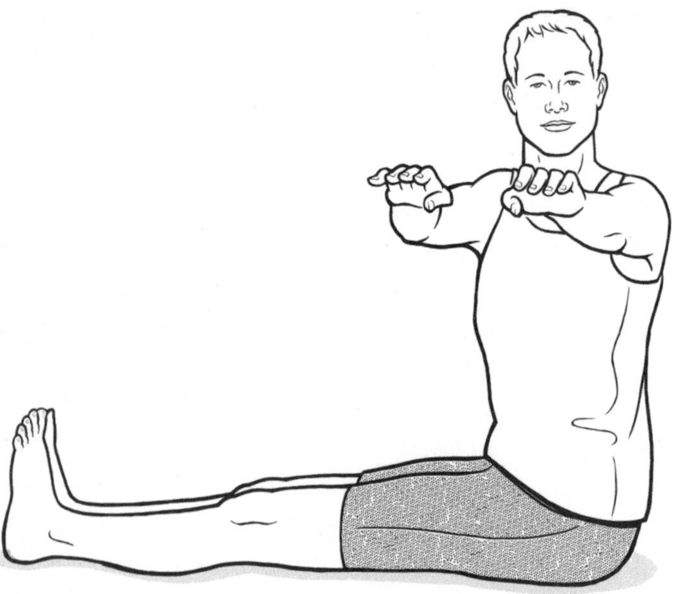

Figure 10.3b
3. Seated Twist Variation

Sitting tall with your legs straight out in front of you, press your sitting bones into the earth and lengthen up through the spine. Raise both arms to shoulder height in front of you and position your hands as if you were holding a beach ball. On an exhale, twist from the core making sure your spine is tall and straight, moving your entire upper body as one unit. Hold your gaze on the space between the hands, relaxing your eyes. Exhale to release to center, then repeat on the other side. End on your hands and knees.

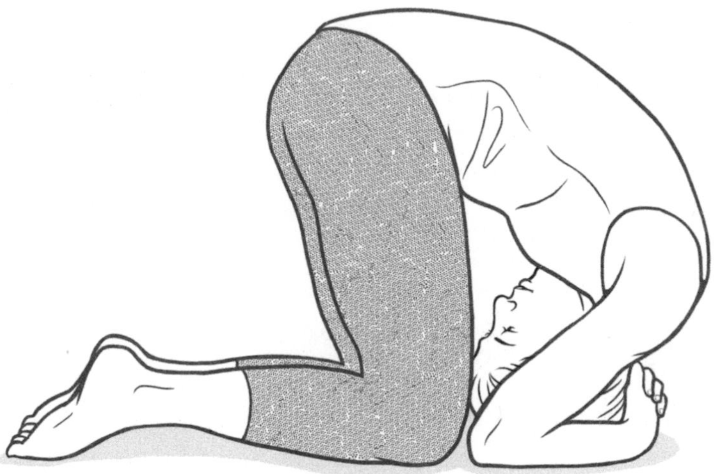

Figure 10.4
4. *Sasangasana* **(Rabbit Pose)**

From hands-and-knees position, raise your hips in line with your knees, thighs perpendicular to the floor. Clasp your hands together in front of you and rest the back of your head into the hammock of your hands, top of the head very lightly on the floor. The weight of your body is on the forearms and knees. Engaging the abdominal muscles, arch your back to the sky. In time you may begin to move the upper body and the lower body closer together, rounding the back even higher while keeping pressure in the arms and knees, not on the head.

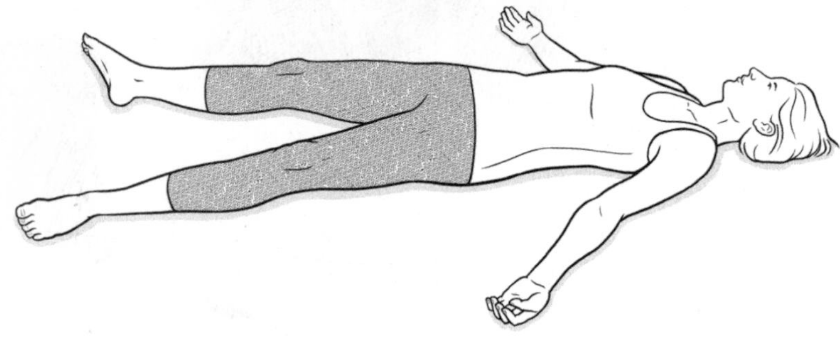

Figure 10.5
5. *Savasana* (Corpse Pose)

You can climb into bed before assuming this posture. Extend your legs out, feet wider than the hips. Place your arms halfway between hips and shoulder-height. Relax your hands, palms up. Perform your favorite relaxation practice. You may allow yourself to drift off to sleep in this balanced, healing posture.

Now that you have so many practices to support you in overcoming resistance, we can look at ways you may further balance your life. The following exercise offers you a clear intentionality to your lifestyle so that you may remain clear and inspired.

Exercise: Life Wheel

How do you manage to stay on your bicycle? You watch for obstacles on the road ahead, steering around them. You shift your weight to balance on the seat and counterbalance your turns. Just like riding a bicycle, maintaining balance in life requires constant attention and subtle adjustments in order to remain upright, with forward momentum. Let's explore some simple ways of balancing your lifestyle.

1. Covering a full sheet of paper, draw a wheel with eight spokes. Include a smaller circle as a hub in the middle. Write your current spiritual intention in the hub. This intention may be a sin-

gle word that anchors you to your higher self, or a virtue, or a habit you are cultivating.

2. Entitle each of the spokes: Body, Energy, Feelings, Intellect, Higher Self, Work, Relationships, and Spirit. Create a personal goal for each of these areas. Remember that less is more. Goals such as, "At least three times per week, park farther from the building and notice nature during the walk into work" or "Reduce stress by turning off the phone two hours before bed Tuesday and Thursday nights" are some examples.
3. Select a goal from one of the areas to focus all of your effort on, until you have mastered it. Then you may decide to repeat this exercise from the beginning or simply choose another area on your current life wheel to incorporate.

Chapter Summary

1. It takes time to change our thinking and behavior because the brain and nervous system have patterns embedded in them. We can, however, change our reaction to the pattern today!
2. View reality with objective calm, remembering there are more response options than simply stress. Stress and anxiety are a patterned response, a mind trick, and not appropriate to every situation.
3. Witness your thoughts and feelings to receive their message while cultivating an objective, relaxed perspective. Emotions are teachers, showing us the path away from stress.
4. Avoiding or resisting our true feelings actually causes pain and stress.
5. Stay present in the process, then the future can take care of itself. Celebrate what you are already doing for mental health.
6. Visualizing situations beforehand trains the brain to accomplish the plan in reality.

7. Anxiety and stress are evidence of a life out of balance. In order to attain balance, consider life as a wheel with many spokes, knowing that there are numerous lifestyle factors you could stabilize. Select just one and do it!

The following chapter views your future without the lens of stress or anxiety.

Chapter 11

From Stress Management to Stress Transformation

We are now ready to move beyond anxiety! The tools in this book support you in releasing the internal patterns of anxiousness and stress. Hopefully your life is no longer about simply managing stress. Through shifting your perspective, you have transformed it. Like all humans, you will feel anxiety and stress, but no longer identify yourself as being an anxious person. If anxiety reoccurs, remember it is an arousal of the nervous system and is 100 percent manageable. Rather than worsening the cycle—becoming stressed about anxiety and anxious about stress—remember that every time you feel anxious it is a learning opportunity. Now stressors are welcome as they are a means to strengthen your connection to the higher self.

Exercise: Experiencing Intention

Throughout this yoga therapy process, you have been working with a personal intention, which you decided on in Chapter 1. You may have refined it throughout this book via your insights and actions. Feel welcome to continue to shift your intention as you learn more about yourself and connect more deeply.

1. Write down your current intention and post it in your work area, places where your anxiety is triggered, and where you rest and play.
2. Set a reminder to pause every day to notice how your internal state is relating to your intention. This can be a time of consciousness, validation, or retuning—some days you will be working with your intention and reaping benefits in that moment, and on other days you will have forgotten it entirely. This is normal; all you have to do is return to your focus. Hold the intention in your heart and enjoy the internal climate.
3. As you follow this process, notice and write down the ways in which holding your spiritual intention changes the feeling or even nature of your daily tasks.

Exercise: Climate Control

Throughout this book you have learned to watch your inner experiences without reacting to them. This internal witness enables you to face normal internal changes. The witness remains relaxed and unchanged, no matter what thoughts or feelings are passing through. Emotional reactions aren't a problem. There is no need to run from your feelings or challenging circumstances. Appreciate the lessons.

1. Witnessing your internal perspectives and feelings with acceptance allows you to explore and get to know yourself. What times during the day do you notice an internal climate of peacefulness?
2. Describe in as much detail as possible *how* you are bringing about that climate of ease. What small habits or shifts in belief moderate that internal climate? What have you changed about your thoughts, routines, relationships, approach, and external environment? Trust that these pockets of peaceful

time will spread like a drop of paint in water, gradually coloring all areas of your life with awareness and peace.

3. Whenever possible, do your best to control your internal weather. When you can't, watch it through the window, knowing you are sheltered from the storm by the true, unchanging higher self.

Maintaining and Continuing

When we feel well, it is easy to relax too much. Small but important lifestyle habits may fall by the wayside as we choose more mindless activities. Just as diet and exercise affect weight gain, if we slip up on our calming routines, we may see a return of the old, disturbing feelings. It is far easier to maintain calm and continue a life of peacefulness than it is to retrieve and recreate it. Should you slip off the path—this is common for most of us, since life is always changing—just accept it and get right back to doing what works!

Process of Change

Change, even when it is in a healing direction, is challenging. It is normal to experience resistance or waning motivation. Think about the last time you tried to change something. You probably thought about whether or not the change was a good idea and how to do it best. Despite this, you probably didn't integrate the change all at once. Typically, change occurs in measurable stages, defined by Prochaska and DiClemente.[2]

The **precontemplation** stage happens before we are even thinking of changing. There is either a denial of the problem or an awareness of the problem with unwillingness to change it. It is okay to be at this stage with some things, especially if we are focused on growth in other areas.

The next stage, **contemplation**, is when we think about the problem and changing it. We become more aware of the consequences of

2. James O. Prochaska and Carlo C. DiClemente, "Changes and Processes of Self-Change of Smoking: Toward an Integrative Model of Change," *Journal of Clinical and Consulting Psychology* 51 (1983): 390–395.

our choices and consider the possibility of changing, although we often weigh mixed feelings about it.

The **preparation** stage happens once we have decided to change; it's time to get ready! We think about what, how, and when to change. Preparation is a planning stage where, despite fear and resistance, we are aware of the benefits of change and are figuring out how to make adjustments. This is an important stage of foreseeing obstacles before they arise and preparing solutions. It also offers the opportunity to envision our lives without the problem! Many people get stuck in the preparation stage. There is fear going from preparation to action. As long as you are preparing you cannot fail, but you cannot succeed if you don't take action, either.

The **action** stage is essential. Learning, thinking about, and visualizing a solved problem will not actually improve life in the external world. Although it is nourishing to feed ourselves the healthy ideas of the previous stages, it is only through action that we attain an integrated healthy routine.

The **maintenance** stage shows sustained action. Healthy changes are practiced and continually reinforced until they become automatic and last for an extended period of time. We are better able to avoid old habits and moments of weakness. It is a "new normal" that brings many benefits, even though it takes time to integrate the change. We may notice thoughts and echoes of the old behaviors but can acknowledge the movements of the mind and are unaffected by them. Effort is still required in the maintenance stage. This stage leads to one of two places: relapse or stable behavior.

Relapse, the recurrence of previous unhealthy behaviors, is common during the process of change. Do not be discouraged; simply revisit strategies from the action stage. Usually, the process will be faster the second (or third, or tenth) time around, especially because we have had a taste of a better life through this change. Peacefulness is not a pass/fail endeavor; relapse can be a beneficial part of change because it teaches us about our habits, needs, and weaknesses. Ironically, relapsing fortifies our anxiety recovery plan! The sooner relapse is addressed, the more quickly it tends to be resolved.

Stable behavior is apparent when the maintenance stage becomes automatic. We have gone to a new level. We have an awareness of a better life without the problem. A return to the behavior would seem foreign now. That former problem is not-self. By making healthy changes, we connect with the experience of ease, contentment, and acceptance, and align with the higher self. The change is now simply a way of life.

Exercise: Maintenance and Continuance

In the world of therapy, there is much talk about a healing spiral. This is the productive counterpart to a downward spiral, where similar behaviors and emotions inevitably lead to rock-bottom. Conversely, the healing spiral is a loop that affirms our well-being. Although similar negative thoughts and behaviors may reoccur, on the healing spiral we are able to see that change truly is happening. Each time we repeat an internal or external pattern, we handle it with more awareness and grace, and it has less impact on our peace of mind. In this way, former negatives become affirmations of change and personal evolution.

1. Witness your own process of change. Choose one area of your life to enhance with relaxation.
2. Make a concrete plan of supporting yourself, then implement those actions. Appreciate yourself in the effort, even if it isn't perfect! Set a time each day to acknowledge and honor your personal aspiration.
3. Mark one month from now in your calendar to revisit highlights from this book. Review and realign your intention. Review the intentions you set and celebrate the shifts you made because of the past month's efforts.

Looking at Your Life Comprehensively

Our view of life dictates our experience of it. Consider the case study of Deadline Debbie the editor, who had a lot of anxiety about deadlines. Debbie's targets were a huge stressor for her because they were set not just for each book that she edited but for each hour of each day. That's a lot of deadlines! Debbie was paid by the number of total words she edited each day—that is, edited *correctly*. Her body rolled forward in a habitual slouch from a combination of computer overuse and fretting about reading fast enough to earn her living. She was thin and often didn't stop to eat properly because she worked long hours to finish a specified number of words each day.

Time in yoga classes was good for Debbie. She started to open up her body and breath. The problem was she found herself in a cycle of feeling good after yoga class and feeling stressed at work. Debbie decided to take her yoga experience further through yoga therapy sessions. It became clear that her attitude was key; somehow, she had to transform her experience of deadlines. The deadlines are a reality—the publishing industry is organized by deadlines. First, Debbie admitted that she hated deadlines and that they were a huge burden that weighed her down. In our Comprehensive Yoga Therapy sessions, instead of overriding the reality of deadlines, we tried to harness the energy of that pressure. Debbie did exercises you've experienced throughout this book. At one point she imagined being on a sailboat with the deadline energy being the wind. She could choose to sail on the winds and move productively through her life. This shift in attitude caused her to sit straight like the sailor setting the sails just right to catch the wind. If the winds (pressures) became too intense, she promised herself to take a short break and refocus. Debbie began to slot time for five-minute breaks throughout the day. She used that time for doing a few yoga poses or taking a short walk outside. She decided to turn off her computer while eating. All in all, she feels empowered!

In your life, as you identify the triggers for your stress, notice that you too are able to create imagery, perspectives, and affirmations that support you in viewing your life comprehensively. As you look at life with new eyes, you can gradually incorporate more practices that support your health and mental well-being. Through the process of guiding your perspectives, you gradually nourish yourself more and more on all levels.

Community Support for Balance

One thing to remember about disciplining yourself to stay in a good routine is to think more about support. The most intelligent or experienced person knows that they will go to the gym if their friend or a trainer is meeting them, but if left to their own devices, they might not make it! Attend a yoga class, find a supportive friend, or contact a local yoga therapist to help you maintain your healthy routines and peaceful life.

Generally speaking, community support is like clothing: some colors look good on you and other colors just aren't as becoming, depending on your skin tone, haircut, personal aesthetic, and personality. It is recommended to get and stay involved with others in order to remain healthy, but make sure the style of gathering matches your personality type. For example, Sami is the anxious type of person who, being afraid to be alone, volunteers for everything the children are potentially involved in. Sami doesn't just attend church but is also on every committee, and time at home is spent continually cleaning, organizing, and attempting to control reality. For Sami, community support and a balanced life would mean attending various events as a participant instead of being in charge.

Conversely, Carol is the type of person who turns stress and anxiety inside and as a result looks perfectly calm. Carol is afraid to talk because it's hard to get the words out around the racing thoughts. Being too close with others creates even more anxiety because of the pressure to say the right thing at the right time. Carol is really good at spending time with just one or two friends. This is a classic introvert. It doesn't make Carol a socially anxious person, it's just a different way of relating to the world. It's better for Carol to associate with smaller groups, which allows mental and emotional balance, and once in a while join one of those committees that Sami should let go of.

Exercise: Customizing Your Community

If you're an introvert, you may seek out groups that let you work on your own while spending time with others. If you are an extrovert, you may look for groups that are collaborative and offer you a chance to interact and share. Your personal interests and causes that light a spark in you can guide you to the appropriate community. Follow the enquiry of this exercise to inspire you toward appropriate community.

1. List a few activities, political movements, spiritual ideologies, and creative endeavors that are important to you or that you have wanted to learn more about.
2. Do an online search for at least one of these to explore how they may be happening in your community. Ask around—you'll be amazed how once you have set the intention the group seems to find you!

Make Friends with Happy People

Everyone in the world who is interested in self-development gathers with others in order to learn and be successful. Yes, every spiritual community, religion, sport, and hobby has a group for support: dancers dance together, readers have book clubs, kids go on play dates, and those trying to develop healthy living habits attend seminars and workshops. You may join a fitness club, go to yoga class, get involved in a temple, join a meditation group, walk with a friend at work, or go to a painting party, writers' group, or quilting bee. Join activities that relate to your hobbies and enjoy being with other folks who also love that hobby. If you like bird watching, do more than just walk in the woods alone—find a group! If you are a hiker or a cook or a knitter or an athlete, find out where there are other uplifting people gathering to participate in that hobby. Whatever your activity, sign up. When you sign up, you join with a community of people who are going to support you. This automatically gives you reason to look forward to an activity for fun. All of the happy people on the planet have this fun quotient in common, be they rich or poor.

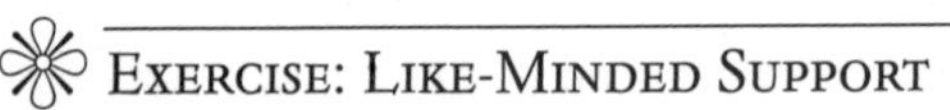

Exercise: Like-Minded Support

The intention here is to give you a long list of potential supports that could be helpful and uplifting. Some days you won't feel motivated to engage in health and live fully; that's when your like-minded friends lift you up. This book is a good resource, but your health-minded friendships will keep you in action. Community is key for us all.

1. What lifestyle habits have you created thus far that are amplifying your sense of peace and confidence? As you think of these everyday routines, list a few ways you can recruit others to support you.
2. Examine the list of groups, hobbies, and activities from the previous exercise that interest you. Who, on an unpaid, friendly basis, will support you in maintaining those behaviors?

Yoga Classes and Courses for Inspiration

There is a saying that "dust falls every day." Sure, this keeps us from feeling frustrated by an unending need to clean the house, but it also serves to remind us of the importance of keeping our minds fresh and clean. Everyday pressures begin to coat us and if we do not make time to "dust ourselves off," eventually we become like the old forgotten mirror, no longer reflecting an image of the true self. Many people liken their yoga journey to peeling an onion: when we work through the current layer, what lies beneath is another layer! This journey of uniting with the higher self is unending, ever more refined, subtle, sensitive, and blissful. With this continuous path of growth, it is important to continue learning about ourselves.

A simple way to stay connected to the higher self and our journey is to find a local yoga or meditation class that suits your level of physical ability and self-inquiry. Yoga and meditation are still fairly new in some towns, so be patient as you seek the style and teacher that best serves you. In the end what really matters is that you have space with like-minded people to experiment with postures, breathing, relaxation, and your own inner world. As long as nothing is performed in the class that will harm you, enjoy what the teacher offers and the overall experience.

If you live in a remote area where there are no yoga or meditation classes available, do a specific online search for DVDs that emphasize your areas of interest, such as "meditation for personal growth" or "yoga for an open heart." Review the feedback and you will have a strong sense of whether or not the product is right for you. You can also borrow audios and DVDs from your local library or download them from an online service. There are many yoga and meditation webinars available as well. Every few months, make the trip to the nearest urban center and attend classes, workshops, and retreats. These brief excursions can go a long way in building and sustaining a rich, meaningful practice.

There are many approaches to yoga and meditation classes. It is true that some classes are going to be a better fit for you based on matching your fitness level and psychological state with the class's aim. All you have to do is enjoy the class for the peace of mind that is intended for that period of time. Turn off your phone. Notice that there are few or no external disturbances. Use the class as an excuse to be quiet and internally aware. Even if you are a yoga teacher yourself, go to a class and simply surrender to the program.

Exercise: Transformation Partner

It is important not to take this journey alone. Through friendly, like-minded relationships you will stay inspired and have somewhere to turn when you need support. The previous exercises have helped you build community. This exercise offers you a chance to explore how to recruit a deeper transformation partner.

1. Connect with another friend or family member who is interested in personal growth. Strike up a conversation with someone in your yoga class. Find a yoga buddy. Like having a workout buddy, you can inspire each other and get through resistances with support. Can you think of someone right now that you could share this journey with? Is there someone

you would like to get to know better, who might have similar ideas and interests?

2. Follow this book and other yoga self-help books together with your yoga buddy and check in about how exercises are progressing. This will help keep you on the path and offers the inspiration of being a support to someone else!

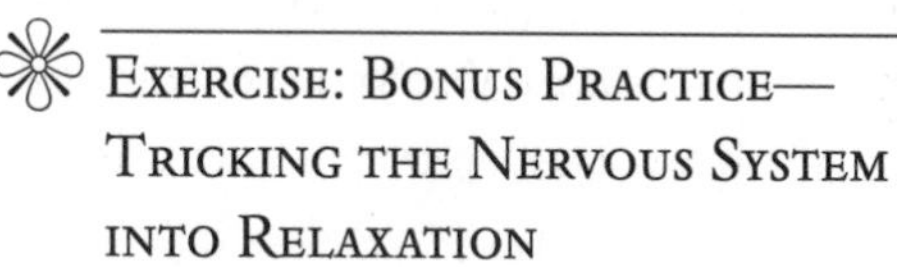

Exercise: Bonus Practice—Tricking the Nervous System into Relaxation

When experiencing profound anxiety, we can use external practices to trick the internal environment. This exercise gives instructions using a yoga sequence, but you can apply the principles to fast-paced walking, holding a Plank Pose, and other activities that increase heart rate. This rapid practice will naturally raise heart and respiratory rates, which anxiety has already increased. (Because of this, as with any exercise program, please consult with a doctor to ensure the level of activity is appropriate for you.) A vigorous yoga practice meets the body in its aroused state, giving an external reason for the elevated physiology. Then, when the internal and external are matched, you can gradually decrease the speed of practice, thereby lowering heart and respiratory rate and tricking the nervous system away from the stress back into relaxation.

Perform *Surya Namaskara* (Sun Salutation) at an exaggerated speed. This yoga sequence is described below. If you are unfamiliar with this sequence, be sure to practice it at a slow pace to learn it properly, at a neutral time, before attempting this exercise.

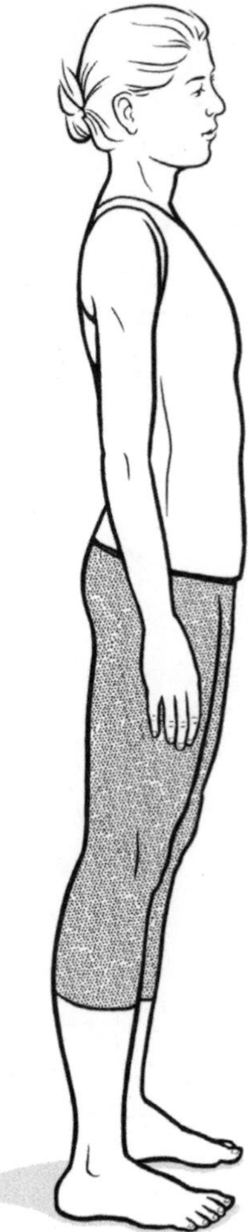

Figure 11.1

1. Begin the practice standing tall in *Tadasana* (Mountain Pose). You can also begin with your hands at your heart in Prayer Hand Gesture as shown in Figure 11.12 at the end of this sequence.

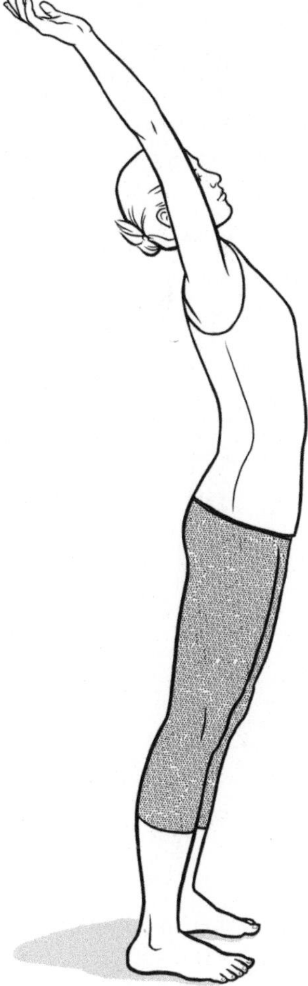

Figure 11.2

2. Inhale and extend your arms up to the sky into *Urdhva Hastasana* (Upward Reaching Pose). You may exaggerate the lift in your chest and elongate your abdomen while holding the lower back stable.

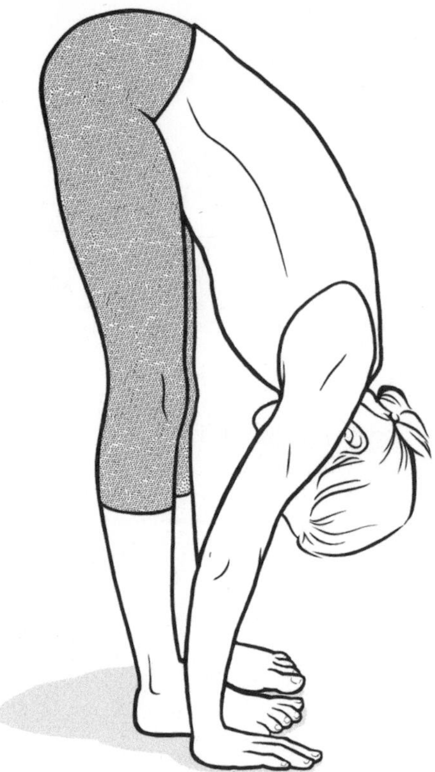

Figure 11.3

3. Exhale and hinge at the hips into *Uttanasana* (Standing Forward Bend), lengthening your spine and relaxing your neck. Place your hands on the floor beside your feet or hold your elbows in the opposite hands.

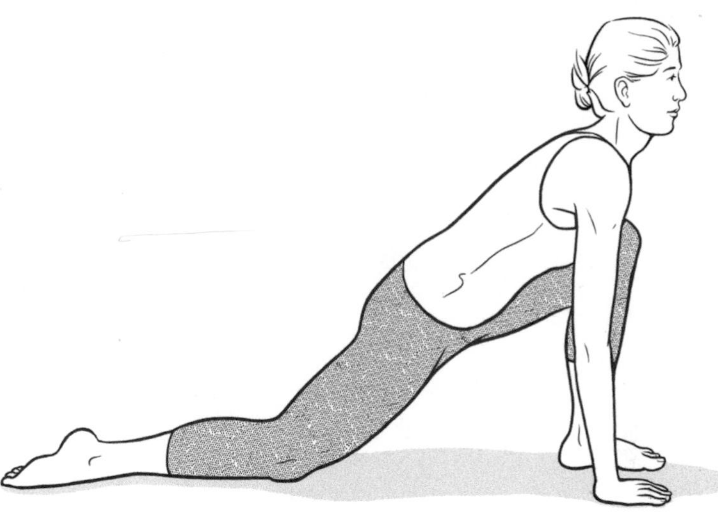

Figure 11.4

4. Inhale and step your right foot back, lowering the knee to the floor as the left knee bends over the ankle for *Anjeyasana* (Lunge Pose). Be sure the front foot is flat on the floor and the front knee does not go past the toes as you gaze forward and keep your chest broad. You may bring both hands to the inside of your left foot for greater comfort.

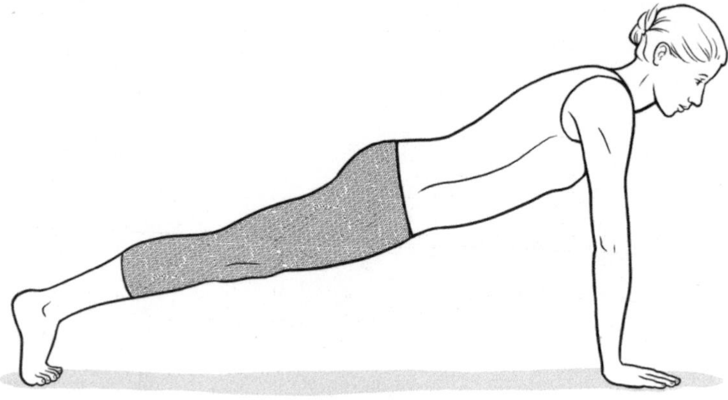

Figure 11.5

5. Retain the breath and step into *Kumbhakasana* (Plank Pose), holding yourself with wrists under shoulders and your back straight. You may be on hands and feet like a straight board or hands and knees in the shape of a ramp.

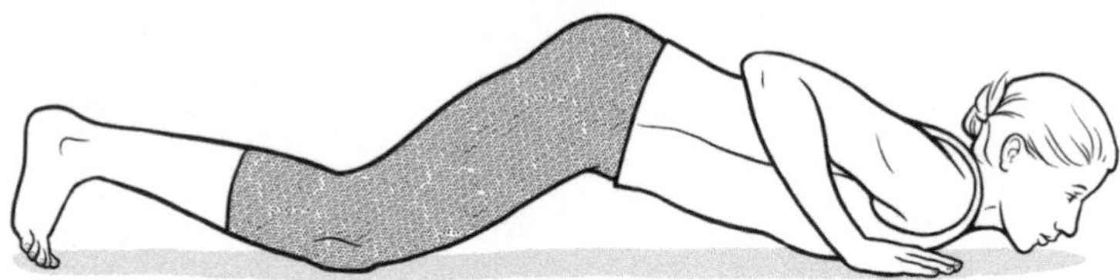

Figure 11.6

6. Exhale and lower your knees, chest, and forehead to the mat, maintaining the straight "plank" back the whole time. Keep your elbows tucked near your ribs through this motion.

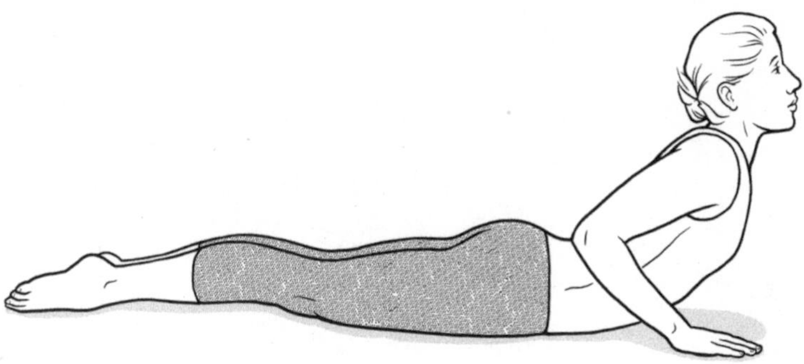

Figure 11.7

7. Inhale, strengthen the abdominals, and roll your forehead, nose, chin, and upper portion of your chest off the mat for *Bhujangasana* (Cobra Pose). To protect your back, do *not* push with your arms.

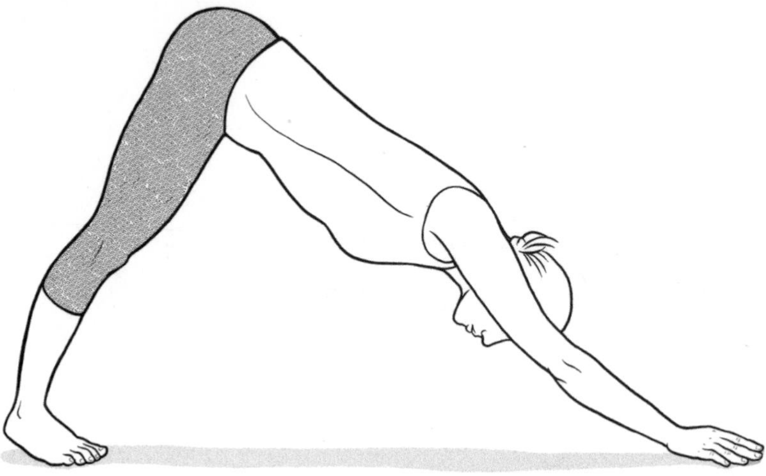

Figure 11.8

8. Exhale, straighten your arms, and lift your hips toward the place where the wall meets the ceiling behind you for *Adho Mukha Svanasana* (Downward-Facing Dog Pose).
9. Lengthen the heels and top of head toward the floor as your fingers spread wide with the entire surface of the hand pressing into the floor. Your body is in the shape of an upside-down triangle. From here, the closing movements mirror the beginning movements.

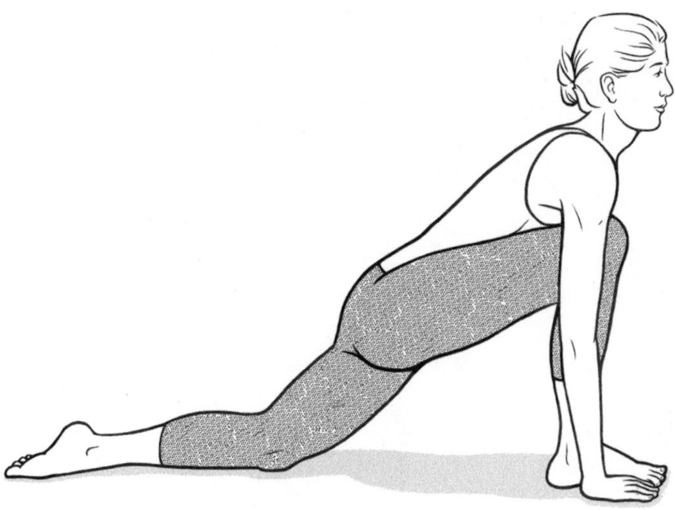

Figure 11.9

10. Inhale, stepping the right foot into the space between your hands. This mirrors the lunge at the beginning of the sequence, offering the other side its turn to stretch.

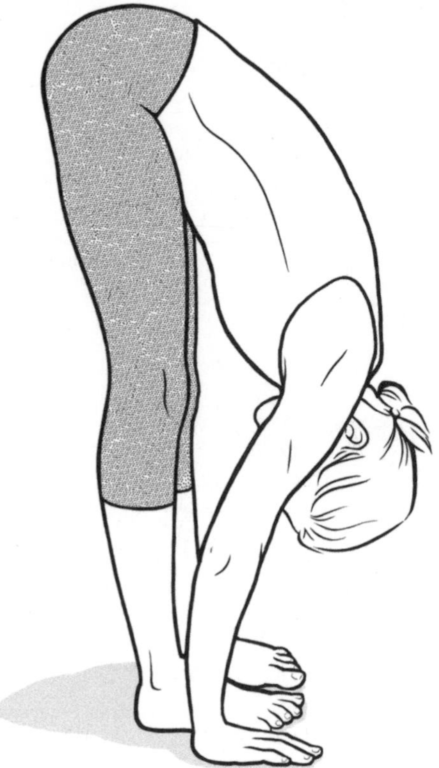

Figure 11.10

11. Exhale and step the left foot up to meet the front foot, lifting your hips and keeping your torso close to the legs for *Uttanasana*.

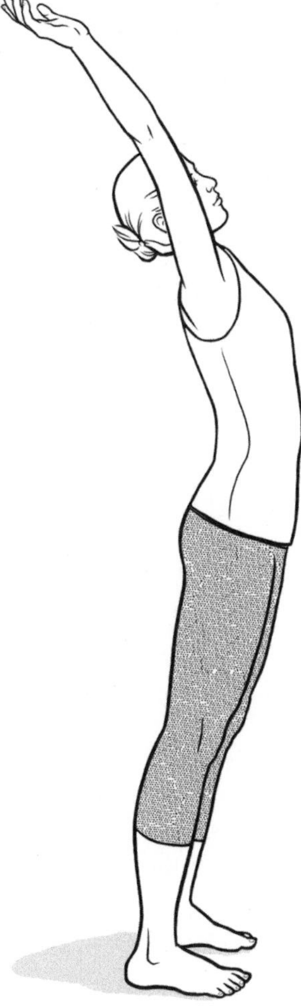

Figure 11.11

12. Inhale roll or sweep up, bringing your arms overhead to stretch up tall.

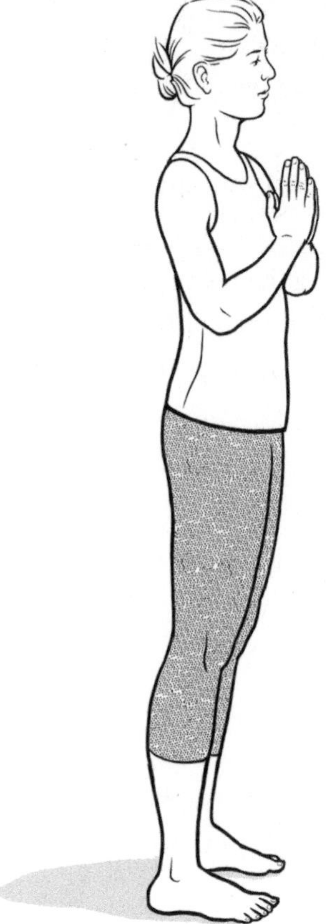

Figure 11.12

13. Exhale your hands into prayer position at your heart center.

Begin to gradually decrease the speed of the yoga posture flow and consciously deepen and slow the breath. Since the nervous system is now responding to the external stimuli of movement, rather than the internal stimuli of anxiety, the physical symptoms of anxiety dwindle. As the movement slows, so do the heartbeat, breathing rate, and even thoughts. The feeling of the anxiety attack dissipates as the body is reset to a slower calm.

Chapter Summary

1. When anxiety recurs, remember it is just a manageable arousal of the nervous system and an opportunity to connect to the higher self.
2. A clear, personally meaningful intention changes the feeling of daily tasks.
3. By combining the restraints and observances with movement, breathing, and mental focus, yoga philosophy seeps into all areas of life, truly supporting our state of confident calm.
4. It is safe to explore your inner world and learn about yourself when you witness and accept whatever you find there.
5. If you fall away from your healthy routines, don't worry—just start them up again!
6. Typically, change follows the pattern of not thinking about change, then thinking about it, planning it, taking action, maintaining the change, possibly relapsing, and integrating a new, stable behavior.
7. Each time we practice a new habit, we handle it with more awareness and grace as problems have less impact on our peace of mind.
8. Our view of life dictates our experience of it. Create imagery, perspectives, and affirmations that support you in cultivating a peaceful perspective.
9. Gradually incorporate more lifestyle practices that support your health and mental well-being.
10. The success of your life is in your hands. Enjoy being fully responsible for yourself.
11. Build a quality team of care providers and community to help you stay motivated.
12. Find a supportive community that suits your needs, interests, and personality style. Let your hobbies and interests be a guide.

13. Join a local yoga or meditation class that suits your level of physical ability and self-inquiry. Even if the class isn't perfect, attend it and simply surrender to the program as it is, enjoying the time for yourself.
14. Ensure better rest so that you are motivated and clear enough to care for yourself each day. Making your bedroom as dark as possible is a powerful shift toward quality rest.
15. A yoga home practice is one of the most impactful things you can do to maintain your peace of mind and confidence in everyday life. Guidelines are:
    - Discover the best time of day for 10 to 15 minutes of practice.
    - Find a place in your home.
    - Begin spending a brief period every day on a quiet self-care activity.
16. The basics of a yoga posture practice are simple:
    - Keep your brain-breath-body connection vital. Remain aware.
    - Warm up your spine in all five directions (upward, forward, backward, lateral, and twist).
    - Sequence counterpostures; for example, follow backward bends with forward bends and what you do to the left side, repeat on the right.
    - Relax at the end to assimilate benefits.
17. Remember, anxiety, anger, and excitement are the same physiological state. Call on your activity or intellect to match the aroused state and bring it back into balance.

Appendices

The following appendices offer you further information about the content of this book. We begin in Appendix A with yoga's foundations in the ancient language of Sanskrit. Appendix B offers some of the rationale for why we selected the yoga postures we did and some of the ways these specific postures relate to helping you remove stress and anxiety. Appendix C gives you information on how to find a yoga therapist, should you choose to deepen your journey with one-on-one professional work. May this information give you greater understanding and inspiration!

Appendix A
The Language of Yoga

Yoga is an ancient Indian tradition. For nearly five millennia, practitioners of yoga have implemented healthy lifestyle practices and deep philosophical applications in order to live in peace. The language of yoga, Sanskrit, is also ancient. Many of the concepts presented in traditional yoga do not translate directly into English. We no longer have the words to fully explain some of the concepts presented by traditional yoga.

In this book, we have translated concepts into English for the benefit of readers who struggle with stress and anxiety and who may be new to yoga. We strongly recommend that you find a book, yoga school, or yoga therapist who can help you understand the depth and breadth of these concepts. While the way we have presented the concepts is completely in alignment with their intended meaning, there are many more subtle layers to their application. The more you understand your yoga practice, the better you are able to weave it into your life; thus, enquiring into the language of yoga is beneficial. A true understanding of yogic concepts supports your decision-making, emotional balance, and lifestyle practice.

Appendix B

How Yoga Poses Relate to Stress and Anxiety

The following chart lists the yoga postures you will find in this book and the commonly held understanding of the associated benefits, especially as they relate to stress and anxiety. Yoga is a holistic system of restoring and maintaining well-being in our five layers: body, life energy/breath, mind/feelings, intellect, and spirit/higher self. Yoga includes a philosophical framework, ethics, movements/postures, breathing practices, sense mastery techniques, concentration exercises, as well as a meditative and higher consciousness. The whole outcomes of these techniques and approaches are greater than the sum of their parts. Thus, it is impossible to list all of the individual benefits and synergistic effects that will arise as a result of yoga practice. We can't predict the state of mind or intentions of the person doing the poses, which dramatically affect the ultimate benefits and outcomes. What we know is that yoga postures, when approached with all five layers of a person in mind, can have profoundly healing and beneficial effects that far exceed what is listed in this chart.

Figure	Yoga Posture	Benefits Relating to Stress and Anxiety
Figure 1.1	*Yastikasana/ Pavana Muktasana* (Stick Pose/ Wind-Releasing Pose)	• Uplifting and helpful with spiritual and emotional transformation • Connected to high states of consciousness • This and any pose that assists in opening the lungs for optimal breathing is fantastic for calming and steadying the mind and emotions
Figure 1.2	*Setu Bandhasana* (Bridge Pose)	• Balances life energy at the throat, pharynx, larynx, and trachea, which may promote clear, kind, and respectful communication • Emotionally this pose will assist in accepting the growth process by improving concentration, relaxation, and courage
Figure 1.3	Restorative Forward Bend	• Quiets the nervous system and the mind, bringing deep relaxation while opening the door to healing • Attitude of nonattachment inherent in forward bends helps you surrender resistance, old thought patterns/beliefs, and release the past
Figure 1.4	*Supta Ardha Chandrasana* (Supine Half-Moon Pose)	• Promotes fluidity in mind and emotions, which helps to cope with stress, anxiety, and other uncomfortable emotions, as well as life changes • Helps improve poise and confidence • Strengthens breathing for greater sense of relaxation and ease

Figure	Yoga Posture	Benefits Relating to Stress and Anxiety
Figure 1.5	*Supta Matsyendrasana* (Reclined Half Twist)	• Due to the action on the spine, helps regulate the nervous system thereby decreasing anxiety and panic attacks, improving sleep and courage, and creating a stronger neural pathway to relaxation • Releases past issues through attitudes of surrender and wisdom • Focus in this pose discerns small self from higher self
Figure 3.1	*Tadasana* (Mountain Pose)	• Represents strength and stability in demeanor, just as a mountain is firm and grounded; emotional and spiritual transformation occur through contemplation of a mountain • Increases sense of groundedness, as mountains grow from the bedrock of the earth • Helps still the mind • Improves mental focus and physical steadiness • Imagine reaching your highest potential as a mountain's peak is high above the earth
Figure 3.2	*Talasana* (Palm Tree Pose)	• Increases confidence through effort and practice of mastering balance (both physical and metaphorical balance in life) • Helps to still the mind as mental focus is required to hold equilibrium in the posture • Reaching the arms skyward is metaphorical of reaching your highest potential

Figure	Yoga Posture	Benefits Relating to Stress and Anxiety
Figure 3.3	*Vrkasana* (Tree Pose)	• Similar benefits to above posture (*Talasana*) • Imagining rooting feet into the earth connects to a deep sense of groundedness and being supported by something ancient and powerful, which brings about a sense of safety and security
Figure 3.4	*Ardha Chandrasana* (Half-Moon Pose)	• Fluidity associated with side bends builds tolerance to passing emotions, no matter how intense or painful • Deep breath into one lung when bending one way, then the other on the other side, demonstrates immediate differences in your energy, fortitude, and balance
Figure 3.5	*Virabhadrasana I* (Warrior Pose I)	• Strong, grounded, prepared hero, as felt through the power of the legs, core, and forward gaze in the posture • Able to face anything that is in front of you with confidence and steadiness • Brings a feeling of firm upliftedness and courage
Figure 3.6	*Ardha Paschimottanasana* (Half Seated Forward Bend)	• Recuperative and relaxing; helps let go of stress and anxiety • Attitude of surrender in forward bends brings acceptance and faith • Quiets the nervous system, emotions, and mind

Figure	Yoga Posture	Benefits Relating to Stress and Anxiety
Figure 3.7	*Bhujangasana* (Cobra Pose)	• Attitude of mastery, includes: confidence, fortitude, power, self-esteem, strength, and perseverance • Strengthens back and lungs, which helps connect to core empowerment • Opening the chest may help release emotions and create more space for joy and love
Figure 3.8	*Ardha Matsyendrasana* (Seated Twist Pose)	• Revolution of spine represents internal revolution, where change is possible • Cleanses spinal nerves by wringing out stale fluids in twist and creating space for replenishment once restraightened; this cleansing represents cleansing in self and life
Figure 3.9	*Dhanurasana* (Bow Pose)	• Changing orientation and relationship of hands, feet, and torso opens mind to new perspectives so creative solutions may arise • Vulnerable part of body is protected by earth while back (sense of support in life) gets stronger; this combination promotes confidence and the ability to feel safe when vulnerable
Figure 3.10	*Balasana* (Child's Pose)	• Posture is reminiscent of time in womb, connecting you to a deep sense of safety, relaxation, and that you are lovable simply because you exist, which takes the pressure off of achieving and proving yourself • Protective, nurturing pose is very soothing

Figure	Yoga Posture	Benefits Relating to Stress and Anxiety
Figure 3.11	*Viparita Karani* (Inverted Action)	• Reversal of perspectives, literally and metaphorically, to shift thinking and feeling around stressful situations and general tone of anxiety • Exploring a new way of relaxing the limbs, which work so hard most of the time; thereby teaching us to relax our hard-working selves more readily • Relaxing for the heart, which no longer needs to pump venous blood back because gravity draws it in this position; this teaches us that we do not have to fight for everything—sometimes relaxation rather than stress is a more sure path to where we wish to go
Figure 5.1	*Talasana* (Palm Tree Pose)	• Increases confidence through effort and practice of mastering balance (both physical and metaphorical balance in life) • Pose helps to still the mind as mental focus is required to hold equilibrium in the posture • Reaching the arms skyward is metaphorical of reaching your highest potential
Figure 5.2	*Vrkasana* (Tree Pose)	• Similar benefits to above posture (*Talasana*) • Imagining rooting feet into the earth connects to a deep sense of groundedness and being supported by something ancient and powerful, which brings about a sense of safety and security

Figure	Yoga Posture	Benefits Relating to Stress and Anxiety
Figure 5.3	*Virabhadrasana II* (Warrior Pose II)	• Invokes the fearlessness, self-mastery, and confidence of a warrior • Open posture demonstrates ability to be loving and generous without compromising strength
Figure 5.4	*Chakrasana* (Wheel Pose)	• Creates a balance between front and back, which is metaphorical of finding a calm, moderate path in life • Simultaneously grounding and uplifting
Figure 5.5	*Ardha Matsyendrasana* (Seated Twist Pose)	• Revolution of spine represents internal revolution, where change is possible • Cleanses spinal nerves by wringing out stale fluids in twist and creating space for replenishment once restraightened; this cleansing represents cleansing in self and life
Figure 5.6	*Poorna Titali* (Butterfly Pose)	• Symbolic of transformational power, honoring all stages of transformation: from egg, to larva, to pupa (including the isolation of going through deep change and the challenge of fighting out of the chrysalis), to beautiful, metamorphosed creature

Figure	Yoga Posture	Benefits Relating to Stress and Anxiety
Figure 5.7 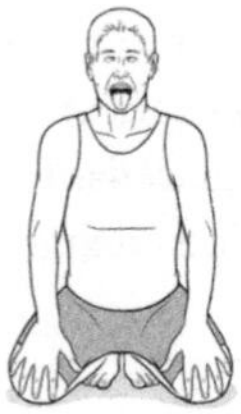	*Simhasana* (Lion Pose)	• Courageous archetype; may study lion social norms for more information • Vocalization connects you to your own roaring voice and the power of your words, facial expressions, and inner strength • May also release stress and anxiety through sound
Figure 5.8 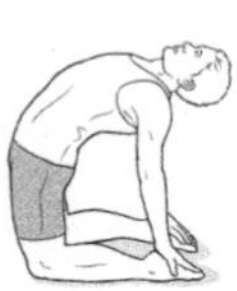	*Ustrasana* (Camel Pose)	• Opening the front of the body promotes a sense of well-being • This posture opens upward, which amplifies the sense of upliftedness and may bring a sense of connection to the joy of the heavens or the fortitude of your own bliss
Figure 5.9 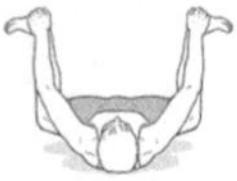	*Ananda Balasana* (Happy Baby Pose)	• Shifting the position of body and the relationship between hands, feet, and face can help shift perspectives • Babies often play this way when becoming more self-aware, and this wonder of exploration can bring a sense of freedom, rather than stress, in life
Figure 5.10 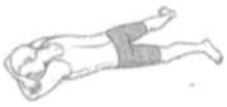	*Makarasana* (Crocodile Pose)	• Supported by the earth, this postures allows for deep relaxation • Promoting a prolonged exhale via the force of the lungs against the ground engages the parasympathetic nervous system and releases stress and anxiety

Figure	Yoga Posture	Benefits Relating to Stress and Anxiety
Figure 7.1	Standing Side Bend	• Opens breathing apparatus which minimizes stress response • Increases spinal flexibility and strength, literally and metaphorically in terms of being self-reliant in your ability to adapt and change
Figure 7.2	*Eka Pada Kapotasana* (Pigeon Pose)	• Helps steady the mind, which can decrease racing thoughts and improve truthful, uplifting self-talk • Promotes courage and self-acceptance, just as a pigeon (which is a breed of dove) will walk through city streets without any shame, meeting its own needs for food, shelter, and companionship
Figure 7.3	*Adho Mukha Svanasana* (Downward-Facing Dog Pose)	• This is the dog's way of saying "let's play"; it engages your whole body for enlivenment and strength • Pose holds within our consciousness the idea of having a constant "best friend" like a loyal, optimistic dog who loves us conditionally • Helps you remember to be your own best friend via this archetype while offering you grounding, strength, and a new perspective of yourself and the world
Figure 7.4	*Yoga Mudra* (Symbol of Yoga)	• Symbolic of our union with the higher self and ultimate well-being • Deeply quieting, stilling, and relaxing posture where there is little room for anxiety or stress

Figure	Yoga Posture	Benefits Relating to Stress and Anxiety
Figure 9.1	*Sukhasana* (Easy Seated Pose)	• Named for its ability to bring ease and happiness, this common, comfortable posture reminds us that we can always connect to the steadiness and well-being within ourselves • Improves sense of centeredness, groundedness, and comfort • Steadies mind and breath
Figure 9.2	*Parighasana* (Gate Pose)	• Beneficial for endocrine system; regulating hormones (especially stress hormones) to limit the physiological habit of activating into a stress response • Helps open the gate between chronic unhealthy patterns and fresh lifestyle routines and perspectives
Figure 9.3	*Salabhsana* (Locust Pose)	• Increases circulation to spinal nerves, helping to improve brain-body communication and SNS/PNS balance • Brings fortitude and energy to the lower back space, which for many people relates to a sense of shame or a lack of personal will; through self-acceptance and assertiveness, stress and anxiety dissipate
Figure 9.4	*Apanasana* (Knees-to-Chest Pose)	• Offers a sense of being self-protective and nurturing/nurtured • Carries a feeling of being safe, small, and held

Figure	Yoga Posture	Benefits Relating to Stress and Anxiety
Figure 9.5	Inverted Action	• Reversal of perspectives, literally and metaphorically, to shift thinking and feeling around stressful situations and general tone of anxiety • Exploring a new way of relaxing the limbs, which work so hard most of the time; thereby teaching us to relax our hard-working selves more readily • Relaxing for the heart, which no longer needs to pump venous blood back against gravity, teaches us that we do not have to fight for everything—sometimes relaxation rather than stress is a more sure path to where we wish to go
Figure 10.1	*Marjariasana/ Bitilasana* (Cat/Cow Postures)	• This pose will assist in creating a sense of inner harmony through proper breathing and balanced movement • Opens the spine and balances the SNS/PNS, simultaneously invigorating and relaxing
Figure 10.2	*Anjaneyasana* (Low Lunge with side bend variation)	• Combines benefits of backbends, side bends, and grounding postures • Brings openness, confidence, strength, fortitude, fluidity, flexibility, adaptability, and similar qualities associated with strength and change

Figure	Yoga Posture	Benefits Relating to Stress and Anxiety
Figure 10.3	Seated Twist Variation	• Increases circulation to spinal nerves, helping to improve brain-body communication and SNS/PNS balance • Steadies the mind; gaze on empty space and this spaciousness is reflected into the inner world, quieting internal chaos and fear
Figure 10.4	*Sasangasana* (Rabbit Pose)	• Introspective and quieting • Helps regulate thought processes and perspectives via heart-above-head position • Offers a sense of privacy and safety to reflect on emotions and challenge old perspectives
Figure 10.5	*Savasana* (Corpse Pose)	• Classic relaxation posture where all parts of body receive basically the same degree of circulation; thus, no area of the body may feel depleted, neglected, or stressed • Archetype of a corpse offers us the time to leave the body, breath, feelings, and thoughts behind and contemplate what is beyond the everyday or beyond our stresses and anxieties

Figure	Yoga Posture	Benefits Relating to Stress and Anxiety
	Surya Namaskara (Sun Salutation Sequence of the Following Postures)	• When viewed as a complete unit, Sun Salutation increases confidence, motivation, and strength on all five layers; it is balancing and invigorating, offering warmth and aliveness
Figure 11.1	*Tadasana with Anjali Mudra* (Mountain Pose with Prayer Hand Gesture)	• Grounding, solidifying aspects of Mountain Pose exist here and are coupled with reverence and gratitude via the hand position; this enables us to connect to the strength within as well as the divine force of nature / the highest
Figure 11.2	*Urdhva Hastasana* (Upward Reaching Pose)	• Uplifting; it is nearly impossible to feel sad, upset, or stressed with the hands flung skyward • Opens emotions to sense of wonder, possibility, and faith
Figure 11.3	*Uttanasana* (Standing Forward Bend)	• Letting go of attachment to dreams or goals • Increased circulation to brain can improve cognitive function, clarify thinking, improve sleep, and support the regulation of neurochemistry

Figure	Yoga Posture	Benefits Relating to Stress and Anxiety
Figure 11.4	*Anjeyasana* (Lunge Pose)	• Assists in opening the entire body as well as the lungs for optimal breathing, which is calming and steadying for body, mind, and emotions • Carries a sense of moving forward with groundedness and preparedness
Figure 11.5	*Kumbhakasana* (Plank Pose)	• Brings a sense of stability through hand-and-foot connection with the earth • Increases strength, confidence, fortitude, and inner fire • Promotes ability to continue with steady breath, even in the face of challenge
Figure 11.7	*Bhugangasana* (Cobra Pose)	• Attitude of mastery, includes: confidence, fortitude, power, self-esteem, strength, and perseverance • Strengthens back and lungs, which helps connect to core empowerment • Opening the chest may help release emotions and create more space for joy and love
Figure 11.8	*Adho Mukha Svanasana* (Downward-Facing Dog Pose)	• This is the dog's way of saying "let's play"; it engages the whole body for enlivenment and strength • Pose holds within our consciousness the idea of having a constant "best friend" like a loyal, optimistic dog who loves us conditionally • Helps you remember to be your own best friend via this archetype while offering you grounding, strength, and a new perspective of yourself and the world

Appendix C

Finding a Comprehensive Yoga Therapist

How Is Comprehensive Yoga Therapy Comprehensive?

Most therapies remove the sting from the client but not the stinger. A relaxing yoga class or session of emotional release eases the sting of unhealthy living. But neither completely removes the stinger. The stinger is usually a materialistic value system that leads to an unbalanced mind. Making healthy choices in everyday life removes the stinger. Thus, yoga can teach a healthy lifestyle that will organically restore health to a person. Comprehensive Yoga Therapists can guide you through the process of healing by understanding the underlying causes of the symptoms or condition.

Comprehensive Yoga Therapy is an integrative process of amplifying and restoring health. It educates and empowers clients to make clinically proven healthful choices about work, nutrition, rest, relationships, movement, and thoughts. These lifestyle factors reduce stress and internal inflammation, slow physical degeneration, amplify the immune response, help regulate gland and organ functions, clear and balance the vital energy, and increase range of motion and pain-free mobility. Yoga supports the entire person: body, energy, feelings, intellect, and spirit. Comprehensive Yoga Therapy practices include movements, breathing exercises, mental techniques, lifestyle education, and personal growth philosophy. These practices help bring physical and psychological processes into balance.

To achieve balance we must consider the whole person and strive to establish health on all levels. Comprehensive Yoga Therapy is a deep practice that seeks to understand the individual's situation beyond the presenting condition or symptoms. It is important to treat each client as a unique person and not assume that two people presenting with the same symptoms share the same underlying cause. Assess each person's lifestyle and thought habits, as well as their breathing, body, complaints, and disposition. By working with the whole person, there is a more comprehensive approach to wellness.

Yoga therapists guide clients toward an individualized comprehensive lifestyle approach that helps them reach personal goals. Yoga therapy does not treat disease and acute illness—that is the role of the medical profession, psychologists, and psychiatrists. Yoga therapists do not diagnose and "fix" what is "wrong" with clients or just treat the presenting symptoms. Instead yoga therapists look at, evaluate, and guide clients toward physical, psychological, mental, and spiritual wellness by restoring harmony and consciousness to all those facets of life. Yoga therapy can have an impact on diseases, acute illnesses, and psychological conditions; however, this effect arises from lifestyle changes, increased awareness, building on healthy habits, and removing ineffective behaviors and thought patterns. Yoga therapy is truly beneficial in working with "chronic lifestyle disease."

Many medical patients, after going through an acute episode of an illness, continue ingesting medication for the rest of their lives. Examples of where this might happen are people with breathing conditions, high blood pressure and other cardiovascular diseases, and non–insulin dependent diabetes. Often once the patient has started taking medication they cannot stop taking it, as the body has become dependent on it. Certain medications lead the body to stop producing whatever substance it was deficient in entirely. The body will not produce substances that are being provided by an external source. This dependency on medication comes at a high cost to society and the individual in the form of suffering, increased cost of medications, medical insurance, and lost productivity. In addition, many of the medications have additional effects that have to be treated with other medications, leading to other side effects. For many people, once medication has been introduced, it is a continual process.

Since the answer to many of these chronic disease conditions is lifestyle change, yoga therapy can make a big difference in today's society and health care system. Today chronic lifestyle disease accounts for about 75 percent of the money being spent on health care in the United States. In response to this, not only can Comprehensive Yoga Therapy help individual clients, it can also save money spent on health care, ultimately changing the focus of the health care system itself. The biggest difference would happen if the lifestyle changes occurred *before* the person's system is affected from the chosen lifestyle, but even *after* the disease has occurred yoga therapy can help. Clients undergoing yoga therapy might not necessarily get off medications, or go back to normal functioning, but there is a good chance that if the yoga therapist works closely with a physician or other medical practitioners, the amount of medication that the person needs can be decreased.

Comprehensive Yoga Therapy works in conjunction with modern medical and allopathic approaches to healing as well as holistic modalities. It is based on the guidance of the ancient yogic texts *The Yoga Sutras*, the *Upanishads*, and the *Bhagavad Gita* as well as modern medical discoveries. These resources provide individuals with specific guidelines for healthy living. Traditional yoga practices are a path to steadiness of mind. By connecting with ultimate concepts and experiencing profound peace, contentment, and acceptance, clients learn to hold a higher perspective through everyday trials. This higher perspective can be likened to a person standing at an overlook viewing a busy scene from a distance. There is an awareness of the busyness, its causes and effects, but the viewer is not involved. As clients gain a broader perspective, mental and psychological habits become clear. Through this process they let go of stress and connect to what is more important. Whether or not there is improvement in the presenting condition, this shift in mental and spiritual state is often reported as the most healing aspect of yoga therapy.

This is *your* journey. Although it is important to find a yoga therapist you click with, what is most important is that you remain self-reliant. Your journey is a bit like training for an Olympic event. Olympians have an entire team of people supporting their path: coaches, rehabilitation specialists, sports psychologists, physical therapists, kinesiologists, technique advisors, and so on. Ultimately, it is only the athletes themselves who put in the hours of training every day to maintain their health and fitness and reach their personal goals. They compete on their own. Who do you need around you to be successful? What motivates you to show up every day and strive to improve your life? Your yoga therapist does not have the power to make or break your healing journey. Only you have that. The success of your life is in your hands.

That said, building a quality team is key to staying motivated to put in your own effort, interpret your needs, and discern where to focus your energies. Yoga therapists certainly know the benefits of working one-on-one with practitioners. However, rather than talk you into searching for a yoga therapist in your local area, let's make this more about *your* needs. This is how Comprehensive Yoga Therapy works: you set the focus. This is certainly to be ethical by only working with those who need it, but a client-centered approach also supports the success of the yoga therapy process. As you examine your needs and aspirations for yoga therapy, your process will clarify, making your sessions more efficient and effective.

Exercise: My Yoga Therapy

1. You are preparing to seek out a yoga therapist. Before you even consider the people who are optimal providers for you, reflect on why you are looking for one in the first place. Write down a list of what you need to work on, leaving extra space for reflection around each item. Think of the components mentioned in this book, your belief systems, psychological understanding, stress at work, relationships, and mind-body aspects such as nutrition, exercise, breathing, and yoga.

2. Review your list of intentions or weaknesses to bring to yoga therapy. Take some time to expand on each need by identifying a method of supporting that need. Can you think of ways to help yourself, before reaching out for more consultation?

The Click

Once you have prepared your personal goals and intentions for yoga therapy, begin to seek a quality care provider. Ask your yoga teacher, classmates, and friends if they have heard of anyone doing quality work. You may also consult the Comprehensive Yoga Therapy website for a list of local practitioners.

Next, do a little research. Review the practitioners' websites and Facebook pages as well as any printed promotional materials to get a sense of their approach, personality, and energy. Call the yoga therapist and briefly state your intention to make sure it is a fit on both sides. Can this person support your specific goals? If anything during the phone call doesn't feel right for you, ask about it right away and give the yoga therapist a chance to clarify. You may need further reflection before proceeding with booking but do not dwell on hesitation.

Go into the first session prepared with written needs, intentions, questions. Your yoga therapist will also likely provide you with policies and guidelines. Remain open to the process of building a rapport. It can take time to get to know one another, and it is normal to feel nervous, confused, or uncomfortable at first. What is most important is that you feel a "click." Can you trust this person? Do they seem to understand where you are coming from? Do you feel seen? Is there a connection? If yes, continue working with that yoga therapist to meet your goals. In the unlikely event that there is no "click," refine your process. First, is it your own resistance or an issue with the yoga therapist that makes you feel disconnected? Are there questions you can ask the next yoga therapist that will reveal their suitability more quickly? Be patient, without being rigid, as you explore the market and discover the yoga therapist best suited to guide you to freedom and ease!

Comprehensive Yoga Therapy Assumptions

- The mind-body complex (*citta*) is the seat of healing.
- Every person is unique.
- Yoga therapy treats the person, not the disease.
- Yoga therapy offers a comprehensive lifestyle approach that complements the allopathic medical model.
- Health must be approached from a comprehensive, whole-person point of view addressing lifestyle, personality, history, and mind-body relationship.

Comprehensive Yoga Therapy Foundational Principles

- Yoga practice routines establish a foundation for change, health, and growth.
- Removing suffering/accepting pain changes a person's inner world and alleviates attachments to outcomes.
- Yoga therapy fosters self-reliance in the client. While the yoga therapist educates, the client is specific about intentions, asks questions, and follows through on agreed goals and practice routines.
- Clients are active students of their own health, not passive patients treated for a disease.
- The five paths of yoga are honored, as each client has an individual approach to health and spirit.
- Clients' personal practice and healthy lifestyle habits establish well-being in everyday life.

Acknowledgements

From All of Us

We dedicate this book to all of our students who, over the years, have bravely explored the therapeutic value of yoga in facing and overcoming their anxiety. We thank them for sharing their wisdom, which contributed to and was an inspiration for this book!

We dedicate this book to all who have nurtured our education and supported our personal growth journeys throughout the years. We honor their unique gifts and contributions with the humblest gratitude. We especially honor The Yoga Institute of Mumbai, India, and all of its teachers, with special regards to its directors, Dr. Jayadeva Yogendra and Hansaji Yogendra. We would like to thank all of the members of the International Association of Yoga Therapists for their dedicated service, work, and support, for their commitment to establishing yoga as a recognized and respected therapy, and for their work in promoting yoga research and education. Our friends know who they are; there are too many colleagues to name!

To all of the Comprehensive Yoga Therapy program participants and teachers for their feedback, dedication, and tireless efforts on behalf of the growing field of yoga therapy, especially Julie Rost, Brian Serven, Nora Young, Ryan Doel, and Sally Sugatt.

We wish to thank Angela Wix and the Llewellyn team for all of their hard work, support, encouragement, feedback, and the professional design of this book.

From Bob

Personally, I dedicate this book to all of my classroom instructors for all my educational endeavors. This book is a manual for personal growth, and the discipline that I was taught in school helped organize the thoughts of this book. The caring that so many of my professors showed is also in this book. In a world where we hear about so many types of problems there exists a tremendous number of positive and loving people. The fruition of all the people who have cared for me over the years comes through in this book. You are too many to name, and many of you have moved on.

For all of the members of the Society of Friends, especially those at the Earlham School of Religion in Richmond, Indiana, where I did my Master of Divinity degree and to the dedicated members of the California Institute of Integral Studies who illuminated my PhD studies, especially Dr. Yi Wu, Dr. Jim Ryan, Dr. Paul Schwartz, Dr. Rick Tarnas, and Dr. Rina Sircar, I dedicate this book.

I thank my wife Kristen and our extended families.

We honor all of the senior teachers at the Welkin YogaLife Institute and the many trained yoga therapists whose comments and hard work inspired refinement in our teachings that impacted this book—you, too, are far too many to name! We love you!

From Erin

I wish to first thank my mom, Donna Byron, for the many levels of support she offered toward my education and dream of running Welkin YogaLife Institute, and my dad, Don Byron, for the impetus to study these subjects. To my brother Kyle Byron, who contributed a great knowledge of science, interpersonal professional relationships, and holistic wellness, and my partner, Peter Arcari, whose insights on spirituality and calm, confident living helped to inspire the tone of this book.

Thank you to the people who have supported my education and healing journey throughout the years, a collective of intelligent, intuitive, caring people too many to name.

Profound gratitude goes out to the staff of Welkin YogaLife Institute, who offer so much inspiration and grace to the community and to me personally on an ongoing basis. Without the efforts of Nora Young, Karen Van Eyk, Ronna Yallup, Jennifer Thorne, Liza Fawcett, Darlene Trottier, Gena Marta, and Jake Mann this book would not have been possible.

From Staffan

I would like to thank and acknowledge so many people that have supported me through the years. I can't name you all, but some people do stand out in my mind.

Among my friends in the US and Sweden: Don Kardong and Steve Jones and their families for letting me stay with them and for always listening to my crazy ideas and sharing their wisdom. To Chuck for hanging in there. To my Arkansas friends: Henry and Jane Hawk for always providing me with a bed, friendship, and good laughter during my visits to Arkansas and Bo and MegAnn Smith for their support and kindness. To the Blackburns for being the Blackburns. To the Bennetts for supporting me and helping me come up with interesting ideas for DVDs and workshops. To Tomas and Maria, to Bill and Elizabeth, to Eva-Lena, Bosse, Anna-Karin, Torbjorn, and Birgit for always take the time to visit with me when I am in Ostersund, Sweden, visiting my father. To Ingrid and all the Nilsson family. We are indeed related!

A special thanks to Helena for supporting me during the process of writing my contribution to this book, and during all the times when I have been busy with all my crazy projects.

Among the yoga community: to Bob, Kristen, Erin, and everyone at YogaLife for supporting me, sharing your knowledge, and allowing me into your family. To Eric and Helene, who run the MISTY conference, for your friendliness and support, and for inviting me to present at MISTY. To Leslie Kaminoff for his friendship and amazing ability to teach. To Sujun for showing me what can be done with hard work and for her ability to combine various disciplines. To Anita Boser and Robin Rothenberg for organizing and hosting my workshops in Seattle.

Among those I have taught with: to the faculty at Nazareth College for allowing me to teach both at Nazareth and on the road. To the faculties at University of Central Arkansas and Arkansas State University, and to Louise, Alecia, Graciela, and Sr. Catherine, as well as others from the lunch table at Clarke University for supporting me and encouraging me during my stay at Clarke and afterwards. To Venita Lovelace-Chandler and the late Fred Dalske for being my mentors. And of course, to all the students who have shared their knowledge with me.

To the Feldenkrais community: to Stacy Barrows for her inventiveness and support. To my mentor, Yvan Joly, who I don't see nearly as frequently as I would like to.

And as always, thanks to Matt and Jennifer Taylor—I wouldn't be able to do this without you guys.

These are just a handful of all the important people that have nurtured me, encouraged me, and helped me along the way. Thanks to everyone of you whom I forgot to mention!

Recommended Reading

Burns, David. *Feeling Good: The New Mood Therapy*. New York: Wm. Morrow & Co., 2008.

Butera, Robert. *Meditation for Your Life*. St. Paul: Llewellyn Worldwide, 2012.

———. *Pure Heart of Yoga*. St. Paul: Llewellyn Worldwide, 2009.

Chodron, Pema. *When Things Fall Apart*. Boston: Shambhala, 1997.

Easwaran, Ecknath. *The Bhagavad Gita*. Berkeley: New Mountain Center of Meditation, 2007.

———. *The Upanishads*. Berkeley: New Mountain Center of Meditation, 2007.

Eifert, Georg H., and John P. Forsyth. *The Mindfulness and Acceptance Workbook for Anxiety*. Oakland: New Harbinger, 2008.

Eisenstein, Charles. *The Yoga of Eating*. Washington: New Trends, 2003.

Emerson, David, and Elizabeth Hopper. *Overcoming Trauma through Yoga*. Berkeley: North Atlantic Books, 2011.

Feuerstein, Georg. *The Shambhala Encyclopedia of Yoga*. Boston: Shambhala, 1997.

Forbes, Bo. *Yoga for Emotional Balance: Simple Practices to Help Relieve Anxiety and Depression*. Berkeley: Shambhala, 2011.

Greenberger, Dennis, and Christine A. Padesky. *Mind Over Mood*. New York: Guilford Press, 1995.

Herrigel, Eugen. *Zen in the Art of Archery*. New York: Pantheon Books, 1953.

Horowitz, Ellen, and Staffan Elgelid. *Yoga Therapy*. London: Routledge, 2015.

Judith, Anodea. *Wheels of Life*. St. Paul: Llewellyn Worldwide, 1999.

Kabat-Zinn, Jon. *Full Catastrophe Living*. New York: Bantam Books, 2013.

Keleman, Stanley. *Emotional Anatomy*. Westlake Village: Center Press, 1989.

Swami Muktibodhana. *Hatha Yoga Pradipika*. Bihar: Bihar School of Yoga Pub., 1998.

Swami Rama, Rudolph Ballentine, and Alan Hymes. *Science of Breath*. Honesdale: The Himalayan Institute Press, 1998.

Sri Swami Satchidananda. *The Yoga Sutras of Patanjali*. Yogaville: Integral Yoga Publications, 2012.

Swami Vivekananda. *Karma-Yoga and Bhakti-Yoga*. Buckinghamshire: Ramakrishna Vedanta Centre, 1980.

Shri Yogendra. *Guide to Yoga Meditation*. Mumbai: The Yoga Institute Press, 1983.

——. *Yoga Cyclopedia I for Yoga Postures*. Mumbai: The Yoga Institute Press, 1982.

Glossary of Sanskrit and Frequently Used English Terms

Aasha: Hope

Abhinivesa: Fear of death / change

Adho Mukha Svanasana: Downward-Facing Dog Pose

Ahamkara: Ego

Ahimsa: Nonviolence

Ajna: Command wheel; sixth or third eye chakra

Alasya: Laziness

Anahata: Wheel of the unstruck sound; fourth or heart chakra

Anitya bhavana: Passage describing all things as transitory

Anjali mudra: Prayer seal

Ardha Chandrasana: Half-Moon Pose

Asana: Posture, physical posture or pose in yoga

Asmita: Egoism

Ashwa Sanchalanasana: Lunge Pose

Aparigraha: Nonattachment

Ardha Matsyendrasana: Seated Twist Pose

Ashvini mudra: Horse seal in which the sphincter muscles are contracted

Asteya: Non-stealing

Avidya: Spiritual ignorance

Ayurveda: Ancient Indian system of holistic medicine

Balasana: Child's Pose

Bandhas: Physical locks of energy in the body

Bhagavad Gita: Foundational spiritual text of yoga

Bhakti: Relationship, yogic path of love

Bhava: Attitude or state of mind

Bhaya: Fear

Bhujangasana: Cobra Pose

Brahman: Unified energetic field

Bramacharya: Moderation

Cakrasana: Wheel Pose

Cakrasana III: Backbend

Chakras: Energy centers

Chandra Namaskara: Moon Salutations

Chin mudra: Gesture of consciousness, palms face up

Chinta: Worry

Citta: Consciousness

Daya: Kindness

Desha: Single focus

Dhairya: Courage

Dhanurvakrasana: Bow Pose

Dharana: Concentration

Dharma: Purpose, duty

Dhyana: Meditation

Dukha: Sadness, suffering

Dvesa: Aversion

Eka Pada Rajakapotasana: Pigeon Pose

Ekapadasana: Tree Pose

Garudasana: Eagle Pose

Guna: Quality of existence

Guru: Teacher

Gomukhasana: Cow Pose

Halasana: Plough Pose

Hastapadangustasana: Toe-Finger Pose

Hastapadasana: Standing Forward Bend

Hatha Yoga: Path of yoga by which self-realization occurs via the body

Hatha Yoga Pradipika: Ancient Hindu yoga pose practice book

Higher self: The true, harmonized aspect of our nature, reflective of our gifts and virtues, which guides us through a life a contentment and calm; could be thought of as the spirit

Ida: The left energetic channel

Ishvara aisvarya: Mastery

Ishvara pranidhana: Surrender

Jalandhara bandha: Throat lock

Janu-Sirshasana: Head to Knee

Jihva bandha: Tongue lock

Jnana: Intellect, realized knowledge

Jnana mudra: Gesture of knowledge, palms face down

Karma: Work, action, notion that every action causes a reaction

Karma Yoga: Path of yoga by which self-realization occurs through work/ selfless service

Kapha: Earth

Konasana I: Angle Pose

Konasana III: Windmill Pose

Kosha: Sheath or layer; five levels of a person

Klesa: Affliction or hindrance of the mind

Krodha: Anger

Kumbhaka: Breath retention

Kundalini: Serpent power or latent force at the base of the spine

Maha bandha: Great lock

Mandukasana: Frog Pose

Manipura: Wheel of the jeweled city; third or solar plexus chakra

Makarasana: Crocodile Pose

Marjariasana: Cat Pose

Marmasthanani: 16 concentration points in the body

Matsyasana: Fish

Matsyendrasana: Supine Twist

Mauna: Silence

Maya: External world

Mayurasana: Peacock Pose

Mind: Also known as mind-body complex; includes the intellect, emotions, senses, body, and feelings viewed as a psychosomatic unit

Mudra: Physical seal created by the body to enhance energy flow

Mula bandha: Root lock

Muladhara: Root prop wheel; first or root chakra

Nadi: Energy channel

Natarajasana: Great Dancer Pose

Navasana: Boat Pose

Niyama: Observance

Om: Primordial sound of the universe; universal creation

Padahastasana: Standing Forward Bend Pose

Pada Prasar Paschimottanasana: Seated Straddle Forward Bend Pose

Padmasana: Lotus Pose

Parsvottanasana: Reverse Prayer Pose

Parvatasana: Seated Mountain Pose

Pascimottanasana: Seated Forward Bend Pose

Pingala: The right energetic channel

Pitta: Fire

Poorna Titali Asana: Butterfly Pose

Prajna: Wisdom, realized knowledge

Prakriti: Nature, physical world, material subject to change

Prana: Life force, life energy

Pranayama: Breath control

Pratipaksa bhavana: Practice the opposite intention

Pratyahara: Sensory mastery

Puraka: Prolonged inhale

Purusha: Consciousness; transcendental self

Purvaja: Archetype

Raga: Attachment

Raja: Psychology, meditation, self-understanding

Rajas: Active, energetic, hyper, obsessive

Recaka: Prolonged exhale

Sadhana: Remembrance, daily practice

Sahasrara: Thousand-spoked wheel; seventh or crown chakra

Samadhi: Union, enlightenment, continuous awareness

Sankalpa: Intention

Santolanasana: Plank Pose

Santosha: Contentment

Sarvangasana: Shoulder Stand Pose

Sattva: Balanced, pure, calm, clear, focused

Satya: Truthfulness

Salabasana: Locust Pose

Saucha: Purity

Savasana: Corpse Pose

Shakti: Creative energy

Shishya: Disciple

Siddhi: Superhuman feat

Simhasana: Lion Pose

Sirshasana: Headstand Pose

Spiritual: Sense of the sacred in the ordinary that can be shown and understood, yet is paradoxically unnamable, intangible, or immaterial

Sraddha: Faith

Sthitaprarthanasana: Standing Prayer Pose

Sukha: Joy

Sukhasana: Easy Pose

Sunyaka: Breath suspension

Supta Matsyendrasana: Supine Twist Pose

Surya Namaskara: Sun Salutation

Sushumna: The central energetic channel

Svadhyaya: Study of self or scripture

Svadisthana: Own base center; second or sacral chakra

Svarodaya: The science of breath

Taittiriya Upanishad: From food to joy

Talasana III: Palm Tree Pose

Tamas: Inactive, dull, depressed

Tantra: Health, energy harmonizing, path of yoga that includes nutrition, postures, breath, and relaxation

Tapas: Effort, discipline

Therapy: Treating the symptoms of diseases; we redefine therapy in the context of yoga therapy to denote healing of disease via lifestyle education

Trataka: Eye exercises

Trikonasana: Triangle Pose

Uddiyana bandha: Abdominal lock

Ujjayi: Victorious breath, partial closure of the glottis while breathing

Urdhva Muhka Svanasana: Upward Dog Pose

Ustrasana: Camel Pose

Utthanasana: Squat Pose

Utkatasana: Chair Pose

Vata: Air

Viaragya: Nonattachment

Vinyasa: Flow

Viparita karani mudra: Inverted action seal (a modified form of shoulder stand)

Virabhadrasana I: Warrior I Pose

Virabhadrasana II: Warrior II Pose

Virabhadrasana III: Warrior III Pose or Line Pose

Vishada: Despair

Vishuddha: Pure wheel; fifth or throat chakra

Yama: Restraint

Yastikasana: Stick Pose

Yoga mudra: Symbol of yoga pose; union with supreme consciousness

Yoga therapy: Holistic lifestyle education to balance the overall human being, thereby facilitating the sacred process of healing

Yoganga: Independent branch of yoga requiring subtle awareness

Yoni mudra: Womb seal, five fingertips placed symbolically over senses

To Write to the Authors

If you wish to contact the author or would like more information about this book, please write to the author in care of Llewellyn Worldwide Ltd. and we will forward your request. Both the author and publisher appreciate hearing from you and learning of your enjoyment of this book and how it has helped you. Llewellyn Worldwide Ltd. cannot guarantee that every letter written to the author can be answered, but all will be forwarded. Please write to:

Robert Butera, PhD, Erin Byron, MA, and Staffan Elgelid, PhD, PT
℅ Llewellyn Worldwide
2143 Wooddale Drive
Woodbury, MN 55125-2989

Please enclose a self-addressed stamped envelope for reply, or $1.00 to cover costs. If outside the U.S.A., enclose an international postal reply coupon.

Many of Llewellyn's authors have websites with additional information and resources. For more information, please visit our website at http://www.llewellyn.com

GET MORE AT LLEWELLYN.COM

Visit us online to browse hundreds of our books and decks, plus sign up to receive our e-newsletters and exclusive online offers.

• Free tarot readings • Spell-a-Day • Moon phases

• Recipes, spells, and tips • Blogs • Encyclopedia

• Author interviews, articles, and upcoming events

GET SOCIAL WITH LLEWELLYN

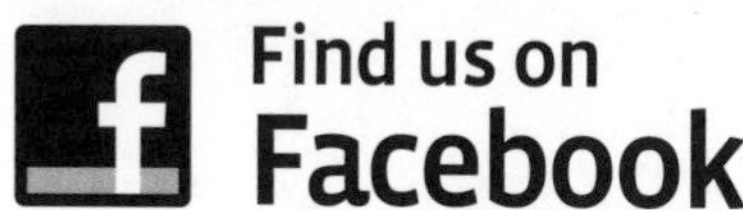

www.Facebook.com/LlewellynBooks

Follow us on

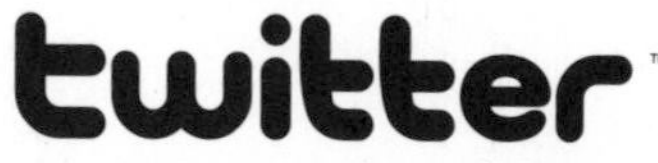

www.Twitter.com/Llewellynbooks

GET BOOKS AT LLEWELLYN

LLEWELLYN ORDERING INFORMATION

Order online: Visit our website at www.llewellyn.com to select your books and place an order on our secure server.

Order by phone:
- Call toll free within the U.S. at 1-877-NEW-WRLD (1-877-639-9753)
- Call toll free within Canada at 1-866-NEW-WRLD (1-866-639-9753)
- We accept VISA, MasterCard, and American Express

Order by mail:
Send the full price of your order (MN residents add 6.875% sales tax) in U.S. funds, plus postage and handling to: Llewellyn Worldwide, 2143 Wooddale Drive
Woodbury, MN 55125-2989

POSTAGE AND HANDLING:

STANDARD: (U.S. & Canada)
(Please allow 12 business days)
$25.00 and under, add $4.00.
$25.01 and over, FREE SHIPPING.

INTERNATIONAL ORDERS (airmail only):
$16.00 for one book, plus $3.00 for each additional book.

Visit us online for more shipping options. Prices subject to change.

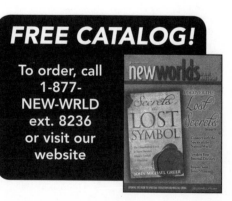

FREE CATALOG!

To order, call 1-877-NEW-WRLD ext. 8236 or visit our website

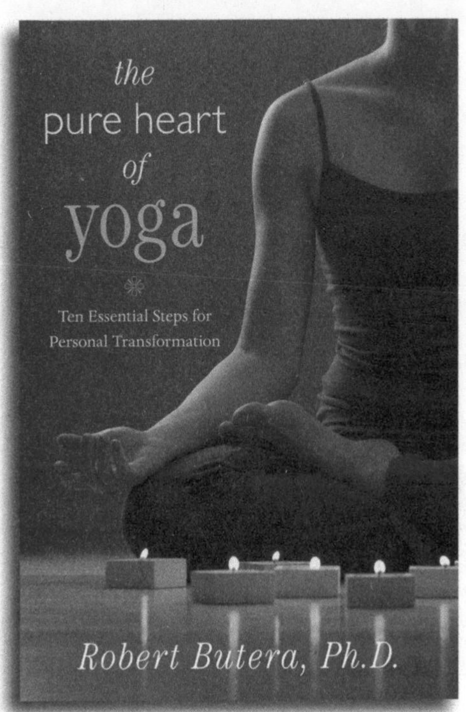
the
pure heart
of
yoga
Ten Essential Steps for
Personal Transformation
Robert Butera, Ph.D.

The Pure Heart of Yoga

Ten Essential Steps for Personal Transformation

ROBERT BUTERA PHD

Connect to the infinite through yoga and experience true transformation on the physical, emotional, psychological, and spiritual planes.

This inspiring book teaches yoga the way the original masters envisioned it—a holistic union of body, mind, and spirit. Dr. Butera's simple ten-step approach invites all levels of yoga practitioners and teachers to deepen their understanding of yoga philosophy and work toward health and self-realization. By cultivating a mindful practice of the yoga postures, you will learn to balance emotions, focus the mind, control breathing, work with the body's energy centers (chakras), eliminate psychological blocks, and create a sense of purpose and peace for life.

978-0-7387-1487-5, 336 pp., 6 x 9 **$21.95**

To order, call 1-877-NEW-WRLD
Prices subject to change without notice
Order at Llewellyn.com 24 hours a day, 7 days a week!

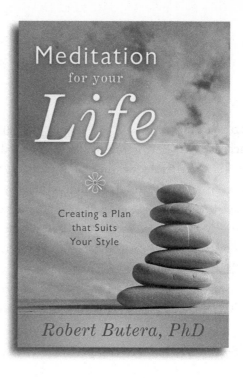
Meditation
for your
Life
Creating a Plan
that Suits
Your Style
Robert Butera, PhD

Meditation for Your Life

Creating a Plan that Suits Your Style

ROBERT BUTERA PHD

Engage in the process of self-inquiry and understanding with expert teacher Robert Butera. All meditation methods are valid forms of practice, but they don't fit everyone alike. *Meditation for Your Life* explains the six basic forms and guides readers in identifying which ones suit them best. Questions and answers, exercises, and journaling engage readers in learning what steps they can take to make meditation (and its benefits) an enduring part of their lives. Wellness and inner calm are achievable goals with suitable meditation styles—using techniques of breathwork or visualization, mantra or devotion, mindfulness or contemplation. Includes special emphasis on overcoming frequent blocks to inner growth.

978-0-7387-3414-9, 312 pp., 6 x 9 **$16.99**

To order, call 1-877-NEW-WRLD
Prices subject to change without notice
Order at Llewellyn.com 24 hours a day, 7 days a week!

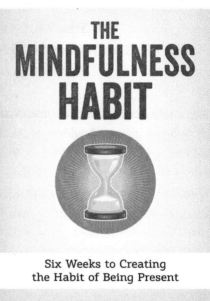

THE
MINDFULNESS
HABIT

Six Weeks to Creating
the Habit of Being Present

KATE SCIANDRA

The Mindfulness Habit

Six Weeks to Creating the Habit of Being Present

Kate Sciandra

This step-by-step book offers a de-mystified and non-time-consuming approach to being present. It addresses the difference between meditation and mindfulness, why mindfulness is important, and dispels common misconceptions about the process. It then takes a step-by-step approach to not only teach exercises and techniques for developing mindfulness, but also includes instructions for finding the everyday opportunities to put them in place. This is done in a way that uses habit-forming principles so that at the end of six weeks, you have both a tool kit and a habit for using it regularly.

The Mindfulness Habit helps you understand the value of living in the moment and offers many ways to create the habit of finding opportunities for mindfulness. In each section of the book, you'll discover information about a variety of topics, exercises and instructions for building mindful habits in your life, and much more.

978-0-7387-4189-5, 216 pp., 5 x 7 **$16.99**

To order, call 1-877-NEW-WRLD

Prices subject to change without notice

Order at Llewellyn.com 24 hours a day, 7 days a week!